Stewart D. Govig, PhD

In the Shadow of Our Steeples
Pastoral Presence for Families Coping with Mental Illness

D0022411

Pre-publication
*REVIEWS,
COMMENTARIES,
EVALUATIONS . . .*

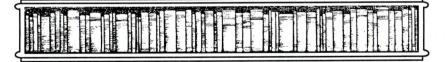

In the Shadow of Our Steeples

Pastoral Presence for Families Coping with Mental Illness

THE HAWORTH PRESS
Religion, Ministry & Pastoral Care

New, Recent, and Forthcoming Titles:

Growing Up: Pastoral Nurture for the Later Years by Thomas B. Robb

Religion and the Family: When God Helps by Laurel Arthur Burton

Victims of Dementia: Services, Support, and Care by Wm. Michael Clemmer

Horrific Traumata: A Pastoral Response to the Post-Traumatic Stress Disorder by N. Duncan Sinclair

Aging and God: Spiritual Pathways to Mental Health in Midlife and Later Years by Harold G. Koenig

Counseling for Spiritually Empowered Wholeness: A Hope-Centered Approach by Howard Clinebell

Shame: A Faith Perspective by Robert H. Albers

Dealing with Depression: Five Pastoral Interventions by Richard Dayringer

Righteous Religion: Unmasking the Illusions of Fundamentalism and Authoritarian Catholicism by Kathleen Y. Ritter and Craig W. O'Neill

Theological Context for Pastoral Caregiving: Word in Deed by Howard Stone

Pastoral Care in Pregnancy Loss: A Ministry Long Needed by Thomas Moe

A Gospel for the Mature Years: Finding Fulfillment by Knowing and Using Your Gifts by Harold Koenig, Tracy Lamar, and Betty Lamar

Is Religion Good for Your Health? The Effects of Religion on Physical and Mental Health by Harold Koenig

The Soul in Distress: What Every Pastoral Counselor Should Know About Emotional and Mental Illness by Richard Roukema

Spiritual Crisis: Surviving Trauma to the Soul by J. Lebron McBride

In the Shadow of Our Steeples: Pastoral Presence for Families Coping with Mental Illness by Stewart D. Govig

In the Shadow of Our Steeples
Pastoral Presence for Families Coping with Mental Illness

Stewart D. Govig, PhD

The Haworth Pastoral Press
An Imprint of The Haworth Press, Inc.
New York • London

Published by

The Haworth Pastoral Press, an imprint of The Haworth Press, Inc., 10 Alice Street, Binghamton, NY 13904-1580

Softcover edition published 2000.

Cover design by Marylouise E. Doyle.

Cover photo by Chris Tumbusch.

The Library of Congress has cataloged the hardcover edition of this book as:

Govig, Stewart D. (Stewart Delisle), 1927-
 In the shadow of our steeples : pastoral presence for families coping with mental illness / Stewart D. Govig.
  p. cm.
 Includes bibliographical references and index.
 ISBN 0-7890-0157-8 (alk. paper)
 1. Church work with families. 2. Church work with the mentally ill. 3. Mentally ill-Family relationships. I. Title.
BV4461.G68 1998
259'.42—dc21
                                                                    98-27119
                                                                         CIP

ISBN 0-7890-0620-0 (pbk.)

For John
and
friends at the Manor

ABOUT THE AUTHOR

Stewart D. Govig, MDiv, MTh, PhD, is Professor of Religion at Pacific Lutheran University in Tacoma, Washington. As pastor of the Evangelical Lutheran Church in America, Dr. Govig served parishes in Wisconsin and Minnesota. He has also taken advantage of many international teaching opportunities from 1981-1995, including visiting professorships at the University of Zimbabwe, the Lutheran Teacher's College in Adelaide, Australia, and at Makumira Theological College in Tanzania. He also was an exchange professor at Chengdu University of Science and Technology in Sichuan, China, during this period. A one-time member of the American Academy of Religion, the Religious Education Association, and the Association of Mental Health Clergy, Dr. Govig has given presentations in Ireland, the Netherlands, Chicago, Los Angeles, and New York City, as well as provided service in many community organizations. His over 25 articles have appeared in such publications as *Religious Education, Journal of Religion in Disability and Rehabilitation* (The Haworth Press, Inc.), *Journal of African Studies,* and *Word and World,* and he is the author of *Strong at the Broken Places* and *Souls are Made of Endurance* (Westminster John Knox Press, 1989, 1994).

CONTENTS

Foreword

As a college student in an Old Testament course that Stewart D. Govig taught at Pacific Lutheran University, I could not have anticipated that our paths would cross again in some distant future. Having spent many Sunday afternoons as a young boy accompanying my father as he took the "guests" of a chronic care facility out for a drive in the country, I was sensitized—to a degree—to the struggles of the disabled, and was thus not oblivious to the fact that Professor Govig entered class with a noticeably atrophied arm due, I surmised, to an earlier bout with polio. An association of Professor Govig with Jacob, wounded by a mysterious nocturnal stranger (Gen. 32: 24-30), seemed altogether apt. But I could hardly have imagined that in some distant future I would be writing the foreword to a book he had written. Unimaginable because the event that would be its occasion had not yet occurred: the diagnosis of his son John with schizophrenia—a far more ominous nocturnal stranger that could, and did, inflict unimaginable pain on the whole Govig family—mother, father, sister, brother, and of course, on John himself.

When the publication of Stewart Govig's book, *Souls Are Made of Endurance: Surviving Mental Illness in the Family,* was announced in 1994, I ordered a copy, largely because a former college professor of mine had written a book in a field and on a topic with which I would not have associated him. After all, I knew him as a Bible professor. I opened it and read the first sentence, "At a convention of the Association of Mental Health Clergy in Chicago, I was approaching the end of my paper, 'Dark Side of the Dream' when, to my astonishment, my tears interrupted the concluding sentences." Of course, I continued reading, and what followed was an overpowering experience of being allowed to witness the labyrinthine journey of the Govig family as they accompanied their son through the valley of the shadow of death. No, he had not died, but the John they had known was as good as dead, for their dreams for him—and his for himself—had washed away. As his father lamented, "the John seated before me will never erase a previous picture of the quite 'verbal' teenager who a few years back so easily met the public in his part-time restaurant job and who posed proudly on a newly purchased motorcycle. Plans for the future abounded. That John is gone." Such a simple, declarative sentence: "That John is gone." Hours and days following, it repeated itself, like a litany, in the recesses of my mind, for my son, too, bears the name of John. An audible "Yes!" came forth from an even deeper place as I read the concluding sentences in which the father, invoking the vision of Revelation, dreams of that day "when not the anorexic-looking, silent John appears before us but the young man we knew before the stranger took his place. Then, riddles and dimly lit mirrors aside, we will hear his story and learn more about God and special errands."

For the authorship of a text on mental illness, there are no better credentials—aside from those of the mentally ill themselves—than those of a family member. These credentials apply to the present book as well—the third in a trilogy beginning with *Strong at the Broken Places* (1988), continuing with *Souls Are Made of Endurance* (1994), and now, *In the Shadow of Our Steeples*. If, in *Souls Are Made of Endurance*, Stewart Govig wrote primarily as a father, here he writes as a pastor to other pastors. Painfully aware that our churches have done very little to support the mentally ill and their families, his goal is to heighten pastors' awareness of the families in their congregations who are trying to cope and not lose hope, and to encourage pastors to overcome their own inhibitions and to get involved. He does not condemn pastors for remaining on the sidelines while concerned, courageous laity have seized the initiative, but offers instead specific, practical suggestions for ways pastors may take fuller advantage of the trust that laity invest in them and of the prerogative that comes with being a pastor, who may take initiatives that health care professionals may not.

Pastors may begin with a ministry of simple presence. From this basis, they may proceed to monitor their own—and others'—stigmatizing language. They may educate and do so, perhaps surprisingly, through curricula that is not trendy but traditional, beginning with biblical stories of Jesus' own affinity with the mentally ill.

They may also become advocates, as Govig himself has become, discovering that the support of a local pastor makes a potent difference among the afflicted families and in the wider community. Not least of all, they may become the receivers, as have grieving family members, of the witness the mentally ill themselves have to give to the strong who are lost in their own illusions of security. Who was it who preached about the man who gathered his grain into barns and assured himself that he had ample goods laid up for many years, only to discover that the things he had prepared were suddenly swept away, in the twinkling of an eye? The mentally ill testify to the folly of such complacency.

Stewart Govig has written another treasure of a book. *In the Shadow of Our Steeples* embodies the insight that, like mental illness itself, which begins imperceptibly with unnoticed signs and portents of things to come, so a ministry of advocacy begins with unremarkable but intentional acts of pastoral presence. Remember the mustard seed?

Donald Capps
William Hart Felmeth Professor of Pastoral Theology
Princeton Theological Seminary

Acknowledgments

Since so many have offered support in preparing this book, I take pleasure in recognizing them here. First, I acknowledge my gratitude for the support of Professor Donald Capps in providing a foreword, and to Marshall Johnson for aid in outlining an initial plan. At The Haworth Press, Bill Palmer and Andy Roy patiently answered final format questions. Editor Peg Marr and copyeditor Karen Fisher enhanced the revising process.

Charles Johnson, Director of Religious Services at the Arizona State Hospital in Phoenix, arranged a stimulating Annual Clergy Day lecture opportunity in 1994. In 1997 Marilyn Washburn, MD, hosted an appearance at Columbia Seminary in Atlanta; closer to home, former colleague Dale Larson did the same for appearances in 1996 and 1998 at Grays Harbor College out on the coast.

I owe much to the expertise and inspiration so freely shared by Jennifer Shifrin of Pathways to Promise, St. Louis, and to Ginny Thornburgh of the National Organization on Disability in Washington. And Bill Vaswig remains a friend with a special gift of listening. Last year marked my participation in a memorable forum on mental illness, "The Haunting Presence" at Plymouth Congregational Church in Seattle. Further around the Puget Sound and in my own Lutheran denomination, I recall similar stimulating adult education ventures conducted at Grace in Des Moines, Calvary in Federal Way, and at Our Savior's in Bremerton, a parish having an unusually good track record in providing congregational hospitality to local residents of group homes.

Along this line, contacts with the ministry of others associated with congregations out of state have become models of achievement for fashioning ideas of inclusion into realities of blessing. I number Bev and Roe Hatlen in Minnesota, Newton Malony plus Susan and Gunnar Christiansen, MD, in California as well as Connie Rakitan in Illinois, the Reverend Margaret England in Arizona, and Susan Schneeberg from Oklahoma among them.

I testify to the goodwill of Naomi Linnell, representing the Division for Higher Education and Schools of the Evangelical Lutheran Church in America. Its 1996 grant helped cover the competent typing services of Carol Bucholz and other expenses. I also acknowledge the ELCA's Division of Church in Society's Disability Committee members, as well as colleagues in its Lutheran Network on Mental Illness.

Here at Pacific Lutheran University I credit Erv Severtson and Ken Christopherson for careful reading of an early draft. They passed along valuable suggestions for improvement. Dean Keith Cooper afforded welcome support, and Church Relations director Rick Rouse made arrangements for me to discuss "presence" with groups of clergy in Portland and Spokane. The lively interest of students in my month of January J–Term offering, "Heaven and Health," stimulated continuing education efforts and further research on my part. I have come almost to take for granted the interest and expertise of friends such as Linda Olson, Mark Winter, Phil Nesvig, Paul Reitmann, and Kaye Olsen. Fellowship with them and other members of our local Mental Health Chaplaincy Board through the years has helped keep the focus upon "chronic" or extended serious mental illness. Thank you, one and all.

I salute John, Bruce and Pauline, plus Ben and Ellen together with the members of an extended family now spread out across the States and overseas. I credit each of them—but mostly Alice—for loyalty and love beyond the call of duty.

Parkland, Washington

Introduction

By the mid-twentieth century, over a half-million Americans were confined to public psychiatric hospitals. An introduction of antipsychotic drugs in the 1950s brought a dramatic change; it set the stage for "deinstitutionalization." This weighty term refers to the establishment of scores of federally funded "community mental health centers," designed to function as alternatives to state psychiatric hospitals. Yet, for the most part, the plan has failed. It was to become, as one observer concludes, "the launching of a psychiatric Titanic, the largest failed social experiment of twentieth-century America." He estimates that 90 percent of the people who would have been in the hospital forty years ago are not in institutions of care today.[1] Where are they now? Some survive alone, and others stay in group homes. Many, however, live with their families. *In the Shadow of Our Steeples* considers deinstitutionalization from a religious viewpoint. In Part I, I invite readers to join me in discovering facts about mental illness. Following a review of the symptoms I seek to draw attention from the psychiatric hospital or asylum-type mental institution to the family caregivers instead. At this point caring builds upon the foundation of listening to tales of their attempts to cope.

"A fine pastor helped us." The brief tribute from a survey looking into clergy contacts with families caring for a loved one suffering from mental illness took me by surprise. The others, it seemed, had cited misinformation and avoidance by pastors. In this book, I seek to help parish-based clergy reduce their understandable uneasiness with the subject. Furthermore, few would blame them for excusing themselves from the scene since human insanity, after all, occupies so much attention from health care, social, and legal professionals. And hospital chaplains minister daily. Thus the question of what leaders of ordinary congregations should do besides has a point.

At the same time, however, parents and other relatives struggle in the shadows with frustration and isolation. They long for ways to counter shame and crave for contacts besides those maintained with health care professionals. By supporting invitations to congregational hospitality and by entering this shadowy arena themselves, clergy can nurture hope in the face of despondency. An opening for new and far-reaching family ministry beckons.

In *Mad House: Growing Up in the Shadow of Mentally Ill Siblings*, Clea Simon depicts the aftermath of madness coming home to roost.[2] In the face of her sister and brother's schizophrenias she must "invent herself," seek help, come to terms with household chaos, and "risk the future." Parents and spouses walk similar pathways. I also employ "mad house" language but with a religious and parental slant. Possibly this book may serve continuing clergy and lay education efforts as a catechism of sorts, a field guide to basic symptoms, treatments, and care models. Echoing them ("catechesis") may lay foundations for a more widespread ministry, including learning, teaching, and advocacy.[3]

Try to define mental illness. The words "crazy" or "insane" will suffice for many and they will simply leave it at that. Throughout this book I deal with serious mental illness (such as schizophrenia, major depression, and bipolar disorder) as including a biological component. These illnesses can affect the brain rather than the heart, lungs, or other body organs. Consequently, they affect thoughts and behavior and often become severely incapacitating and long term.[4]

While "mental" also suggests spirit or soul, plus the noble activities of reason and intellect, "illness" underscores loss. It can suggest a forfeiture of health, or perhaps loss of a job or customary social contacts. Add those anxious hopes for treatment success and cure to the mix. Eventually, getting acquainted with medical and social treatment systems may become necessary. Combining "mental" with "illness," then, invites complicated connections; it actually involves a task more than a concept.

I take on this effort and seek to lead readers beyond discomfort with mental illness. It means investigating current "insanity" talk from a layperson's viewpoint besides studying proven avenues of support for those already occupied with the burdens of mental stresses. In *Souls Are Made of Endurance: Surviving Mental Illness in the Family,*[5] I make an autobiographical start. Here is the story of a parent who encounters—for some twenty years—life together with a son diagnosed as suffering from major mental illness symptoms. His mother, siblings, and I are still "consumers" of mental health services in this country. I claim no authority as a mental health professional in discussing these affairs; rather, I represent the *informal* caregiver too often overlooked in the health care system. And always in my thoughts are narratives of other family members so engrossed.

The wide acceptance of medical language for heart disease and cancer in church circles suggests an eventual opening for this subject's parlance as well. But the public's indifference plus its exaggerations and ridicule raise barriers against it. And they only grow higher with TV depictions of courtroom "insanity" pleas and an edge of fear lying just outside polite conversations about serious mental illness. Thus, the chapters of Part I (Listener) also invite learners to counter misgivings with wider information. Family dynamics here are meant not as a hint for efforts at exorcism and cure; rather, they are offered to promote an onlooker presence from those sympathetic enough to notice.

"Presence" has many contexts. Its roots run deep, back to Israel's wilderness sojourn in Sinai and to subsequent political and spiritual crises. But the Shekinah (the presence of God) continued also for the long run, and for the more mundane, perennial crunch times as well:

> Remembering the Ark of the Covenant which moved with the people, Israel always talked about God's dwelling "in the midst of the people of Israel" (Ezekiel 43:7). That is why Israel could sense the nearness of his Shekinah even in exile. . . . In place of the ruined temple in Jerusalem, Israel had the sabbath as a "place in time." The presence of God in space is transferred to his presence in time.[6]

Christians will treasure times recalling our Lord's promise, "Where two or three are gathered, there am I in the midst" (Matt. 18:20),[7] and for generations have hushed themselves before Table and Altar Presence. Furthermore, believers can strive to love one another better (John 15:12) in hard times and thus "be there" for others with courage to care.

Families facing continuing symptoms of mental disorder will welcome in particular the pastor willing to surprise them by asking about the dashed plans, dead-end care initiatives, and humiliation; they will thank God when the pastor decides to network them with other floundering neighbors in church or simply to accompany them through the foggy steps of trying once more. When words fail in acute or crisis times, they can still take root in the more distant chronic background. Stories can inform and move others to take note. They can also uncover prejudice and falsehoods. Hence, the analysis of Part II (Mediator) argues for putting newfound insights to work in preaching and teaching. Carefully planned give-and-take sessions promise success in changing public attitudes toward acceptance and respect. In Part III (Advocate), I apply tried models for service and ministry. Some congregations and other groups are already leading the way. These champions in the cause can help the rest of us discover new avenues for advocacy. The final chapter, "Habits of Presence," reverses an order of things: ministry *from* the ones hearing voices in silent apathy is a blessing to caregivers today who trust in the power of our Lord's presence "to the end of the age" (Matt. 28:20).

Many clergy operate with tight schedules. Not every priority gets deserved attention. Thus, what is written here should be taken as a response to the challenge presented from a nonaccusatory stance. Furthermore, I agree with a caregiver colleague who has said that program organizers should take care that "a large sack of frustrations and demands for immediate restitution are not suddenly dumped on the desk of the clergy or lay leader."[8] In these reflections I seek to formulate an interpretive framework to add to those offered by psychology, social work, and medicine. It includes a description of mental disorder and reference to revolutionary medical treatments recently undertaken. The high incidence of personal suffering involved in this illness also points to several ongoing social consequences of deinstitutionalization: welfare costs, homelessness, and overcrowded jails.

Several current texts clarify how family members may adapt better to persistent mental illness in their midst. One book offers comfort to the children, siblings, and partners of loved ones grappling with this ailment by seeking to break barriers of social isolation. Profuse listings of sources for information and support would assure them that they need not feel there is "nowhere to turn" in times of despair or frustration.[9] But places of refuge available through a religious congregation or its leadership are not even mentioned in its pages. Another book registers the "coping resources" of friends, support groups, and an advocacy organization such as the National Alliance for the Mentally Ill (NAMI). The word "clergy" appears on one page, but that is all: no further reference whatsoever informs the reader who may ask "How?" at this point.[10]

LeRoy Spaniol, Cheryl Gagne, and Martin Koehler have recently edited *Psychological and Social Aspects of Psychiatric Disability*.[11] Of its sixty-five selected essays, only one concerns the religious resource area and it ventures a broad vision: "Spirituality and Serious Mental Illness." Harriet Lefley's volume, *Family Caregiving in Mental Illness,* presents impressive historical and life cycle sensibilities.[12]

Treat *In the Shadow of Our Steeples* as a text seeking mostly to fit parish-based clergy, lay professionals, and their congregations into this scene. I do not dismiss the good work already undertaken; may it only prosper and expand. Yet, I still pursue further innovative and practical ways Christian leaders may learn to teach and guide congregations away from public stigma toward a *ministry of presence*. More fine pastors have much yet to offer members of society's "lunatic fringe" and to those who love them.

I also invite others who are just beginning their acquaintance with this seldom acknowledged caregiving to join our extended family in continuing efforts to educate ourselves and others. Together we can move on to advocate acceptance and better attitudes about neighbors struggling with clinical depressions, schizophrenias, and bipolar disorders. Advocacy will offer another way to "bear one another's burdens" (Gal. 6:2).

In locating the family pain surrounding these marginalized and despised citizens, an unexpected vision may dawn. A more subtle but enriched practice of Christian love—as defined by the humbled and defeated themselves—can transform our obsessions with success and cure into the surprising joys of surrender to the One who offers peace (John 20:26).

PART I: LISTENER

We have forty board and care homes in our area.
Ten of them are in the shadow of our steeple.

The Reverend Joseph W. Alley
Caring Congregations

Chapter 1

The Challenge

One in every five Americans will have a mental disorder at some time in life.

Lewis L. Judd, MD
National Institutes of Mental Health

Schizophrenia is a common condition. It attacks one person in every 100 in all types of society and culture the world over. Yet it remains shrouded in secrecy, ignorance and fear.

Gwen Howe
The Reality of Schizophrenia

For the first time a young pastor had encountered mental illness in the congregation he served. "I attempted to minister to a young woman who suffered from schizophrenia," he recalled, but "lacking the needed knowledge at the time about this illness . . . I am sure I did little more than provide a ministry of presence."[1]

Yet by comparison to the denial, avoidance, and feelings of powerlessness among so many of his clergy colleagues, he had actually begun a foundation for ministry. *He had made himself present.* In what follows I will seek to explore his modest claim of attention to the woman's illness and thereby, indirectly, to the situation of her family as well. I will also address the hint for more direction and support in his pastoral initiative.

This will require first of all an overview of the shrouded realities of mental disorder and how the illness manifests itself.

BREAKDOWNS IN THE SUFFERER

People who depart from norms of behavior set down by the majority make us uneasy. Inside, we conclude they have crossed the line. Sometimes, in public, we label them as abnormal ("nutty") and feel threatened in a vague way. This even happened to Jesus in his home at Capernaum. When he caused a commotion there his family tried to restrain him, for people were saying he was "beside himself" or mad (Mark 3:19b-27). A similar episode happened to the Apostle Paul. After this missionary to the Gentiles' speech before Festus, the Roman procurator burst out with the charge, "Paul, you are out of your mind; your great learning is turning you insane" (Acts 26:24-29). Subsequent events vindicate both our Lord and his Apostle but issues related to such personal and public tensions remain. Who always sees the truth clearly? Sometimes could it even be the one made out as the "threat"? The fine line between a creative emotional experience and an abnormal one keeps moving, it seems, and is difficult to pin down.

But mental illness is different from the social deviance illustrated above. It refers to long-lasting disturbances of an individual's thinking, mood, or behavior. Most of us have sensed periods of depression, vague fears, or outbursts of speech and behavior that make for uneasy thoughts afterward. But when the stages persist and interfere with daily living, such episodes can become symptomatic and infer something deeper. Persons who may simply appear to be dissatisfied, unhappy, or social misfits are not what I mean. Why try to cast everyday pains of living as diseases to be cured? Mental illness will strike deeper and limit one's ability to converse with family and friends, interview for a job, get along with co-workers or perform certain duties as, for example, those of a student.[2]

At college when Bill found himself unable to study he would go out for long walks. But away from the campus he began to look over his shoulder because of the seven-foot-tall beings he sensed were following along the trail. By his senior year the ghosts had also pursued him to class. In addition, their voices were now audible. "Those times were scary," he recalls, but "then I also started getting scared going to the cafeteria to eat. . . . I kept up my grades, but I had this other life." Bill was suffering not only from false impressions, but from bizarre delusions completely resistant to reasoned argument. Bill's "unwellness" pushed him toward a life of chaos and pain. When another student failed to make it for a final exam, he composed a letter to explain:

Dear Professor Smith:

I know I should have talked with you earlier, but this is extremely difficult to talk about, hence this letter. This last spring semester I took a medical leave of absence related to a generalized panic disorder. I have been working with a psychologist . . .

Sometimes—a lot of the time—the consequences of not keeping up on my studies can get wildly irrational and exaggerated in my mind . . . leading to nightmares, panic attacks, insomnia, sweating, tearfulness, hyperventilation, difficulty swallowing, and suicidal ideation (I have made a commitment and contract to not do this).

Sometimes I feel like Job in the Bible . . . I think God strikes me with lightning when the panic attacks cause a literal electrical sensation through my body. I want to change this because this is terrorizing me and I'm exhausted.

What's important to me is not to lose respect from others since the extent of my relationships are distant and loss is increasingly more painful.

I need to know Hope. . . . I have told you probably more than you want to know but it explains something of my inconsistency. I need to pass your course. (I also needed to unload my crazy head.)

Zachary[3]

A young woman, Carol, described her journey into mental illness:

One night I was awakened by a man calling my name. A powerful presence filled my bedroom. I opened my eyes. There was Jesus, standing over me, right next to my bed. Next to Jesus, I felt so minuscule. . . . I wasn't ready for Him yet. I

was too weak. "Go away," I said, pulling the covers over my head.
Then came the voices:
"Be good."
"Do bad," a second speaker advised.
"Stand up," came the command.
"Sit down," countered another.
I was confused.[4]

Overacuteness of the senses and distortions of visual stimuli are common: the color red becomes a glowing scarlet and a dog takes on the appearance of a tiger. Auditory hallucinations are by far the most common of these false sensations. A single voice intrudes with, "Why not?" or "Be it." Choirs will sing. In the vast majority of cases the communication is unpleasant. Voices accuse and revile a person for past misdeeds.[5]

An energetic and effective pastor began making a series of poor judgments and bad decisions in his ministry. Trusted friends raised serious questions. His medical doctor diagnosed high blood pressure as the cause of a three-week-long headache. Sternly, she advised her patient to reduce at once his outer stress load. "But it didn't matter," the pastor remembered, "I didn't care much about anything. I had no sense of what had happened to me." The time-tested skills of making small talk, masking feelings, and pushing toward success were left behind. It was time to enter the hospital for treatment of depression.[6]

With Bill, Carol, and the pastor, the stimuli of skewed senses, delusions, and hallucinations produced an altered sense of self. This, in turn, led to a "nervous breakdown," the popular explanation for abrupt and dramatic changes in emotions, movements, and behavior.[7] Defining breakdown today as disease (and thereby linking it to medical measurement of body physiology) may ease the awful transits from the despair delusions generate to welcome prospects for effective treatment. But medical "disease talk" tends to objectify experience. We invoke science and try to stand apart; thereupon we lean toward presuming an eventual control and favorable outcome through medical attention from our "Medical Dieties." Real life situations, however, must also deal with healing and cure postponements and with individual and subjective states of personal feelings, that is, with lingering disease or unwellness. Illness, Arthur Frank reminds us, can live on and on through the disease; illness talk begins where medicine (disease) discussion leaves off and admits to actualities of horror and frustration of a body breaking down. "Illness talk is a story about moving from a comfortable body to one that forces me to ask: What's happening to *me*? Not *it*, but *me*."[8] And the question often ushers with it the companion query: Why? It can only beckon us to look for answers more urgently. From the challenges of breakdowns in the sufferers we join the search for more effective treatment and assume "it" will all some day carry only frightening memories.

ELUSIVE SYMPTOMS FOR THE CAREGIVERS

Each of the sufferers cited above were being brought to their knees by happenings beyond their control. At times restless and agitated, there was even a danger they might hurt themselves or others, especially if the "voices" told them to. Hopefully if Bill and Carol were to follow the pastor's example, they too would have been persuaded to enter a hospital. Its locked "psycho" ward might have been required for a short time because in this refuge trained mental health professionals would get a chance to observe—in a controlled setting—the presence of various symptoms.

Therapy

Several behavioral characteristics from a baffling array would likely have arisen in each case. "Mental illness" itself involves disputable characteristics and debatable boundaries. It is generally agreed that most psychiatric diagnoses are less definitive than diagnoses in general physical medicine. Observers will note excessive elation or profound unhappiness, for example, and a given mood can sometimes blend with another. We could add signs of personality changes, difficulty sleeping, withdrawal, and unusual fearfulness (paranoia) to the diagnostic list. Furthermore, a trained mental health professional may wish to mark a degree of severity in the atypical behavior presenting itself—mild, moderate, or severe. Clinical interviews and psychological testing, plus surveys of social and personal histories, will follow.[9] And in the search for a truthful diagnosis—similar to a biblical prophet's—some degrees of "mental illness" will be discovered by the caregiver's art.

A set of observations forming a pattern of behavior—symptoms and syndromes—may provide enough data over the course of weeks, months, or years for professionals to discover what they term affective disorders, schizophrenia, anxiety disorders, or dementias.[10] The basis for a formal intervention emerges.

Talk therapy, self-help groups, and—sometimes in cases of severe depression—electroconvulsive therapy (ECT) may come next. Assuming along with many experts, however, that mental disorders arise in part from biological factors involving the brain (in contrast to bad habits, weakness of will, or bad parenting) medication will frequently take precedence over such psychodynamic and behavioral models of treatment.

Common medication drugs have included Thorazine, Prolixin, Haldol, and Navane. These and other neuroleptics help relieve hallucinations, delusions, and thought disorders since they appear to correct imbalances in the chemicals acting to help brain cells communicate with each other. Sometimes this therapy will become remarkably effective. As happens in the case of other medications such as penicillin, doctors are thereby able to lessen and control illnesses even when they cannot cure them, that is, remove every symptom.[11]

Meanwhile, families gradually recognize the seriousness of these events. They place faith and hope in professional caregivers because they are the ones among us expected to know the answers. Still, "If family members encounter professionals who maintain that families are responsible for the illness, then family members will have a double burden, because their worst fears seem to be confirmed by an expert."[12] Professional/family relations need improvements in communication for a common agenda of care.

Rehabilitation

Jess, a college student like Bill, suffered a similar collapse. When things eventually fell apart, he dropped out of school but chose to hang out with friends in an apartment near the campus. Yet not even their acceptance and friendship could calm things down. Anxieties multiplied. Next came hospital treatment lasting several months. Today, however, the young man boasts not only a bachelor's degree but a master's degree as well. A promising career beckons him to get on with his life. The sufferer was cured. "But," Jess warns, "there's such a fine line between sickness and wellness."

People can and do recover from mental illness. Others, however, will live with symptoms more or less under control; how well such persons will function in society depends a great deal upon community support. As therapy evaluates symptoms and possible causal roots and follows up with talk and chemotherapy *cure*, so rehabilitation seeks to *restore*. This means caregivers turning away from a client's illness liabilities and moving more toward that person's strengths and assets. Hopefully treatment and restoration can even occur at the same time or at least in close sequence. Caregivers also appear from the "helping professions": case managers, nurses, psychologists, administrators, and others. To reinstitutionalize persons with severe psychiatric problems following the deinstitutionalization of the 1960s is cost prohibitive. Thus an ideal rehabilitation will "assist persons with long-term psychiatric disabilities [to] increase their functioning so that they are successful and satisfied in the environment of their choice with the least amount of ongoing professional intervention."[13] Such environments may involve partly supervised house or apartment dwellings, fully supervised group-home residences, or support group settings sponsored by a local mental health center. There will be skills teaching and sometimes classes at community college or university. How to interview for a job, make conversation, program a computer, and respond to someone else's feelings will be topics on the program.

For some, the road is long. Hope will flicker at relapse times. Furthermore, people who are chronically ill sometimes find their social support (including church) evaporating at a time when they need it the most. Family and friends may become anxious and ill at ease around them, never knowing quite what to say or do. Meanwhile the professional helpers will strive to restore their clientele by cultivating patience. They will seek new technology, and never abandon a vision to rehabilitate in some measure, however modest.

Always in the background lurks the task of trying somehow better to manage stigma.

It goes all the way back to David in the Psalms, doesn't it?

> I have passed out of mind like one who is dead; I have become like a broken vessel. For I hear the whispering of many—terror all around!— As they scheme together against me, as they plot to take my life. (Psalm 31:12-13)

THREATENING IMPRESSIONS TO THE PUBLIC

The sufferings of Carol and Bill began as intensely personal and private events. Yet as they never gave up trying to get better, in due time Madeleine L'Engle's remark about inner trials could have described spiritual rebirth for them:

> It is when things go wrong, when the good things do not happen, when our prayers seem to have been lost, that God is more present. We do not need the sheltering winds when things go smoothly. We are closest to God in the darkness, stumbling along blindly.[14]

Jess had also stumbled and heard voices. Through treatment and rehabilitation, however, he had kept them at bay; eventually they disappeared and he was healed. Faith even grew in L'Engle's picture of darkness. But its lurking gloom was mostly hidden except from persevering caregivers, close relatives, and friends who had begun to share it with Jess. As a professional leader of a congregation, however, the illness stresses in the case of the pastor cited previously had become disturbingly apparent to co-workers. He would have to "go public" with his illness. What happens then? The stage is set for stigma's path toward misunderstanding and injustice.

Screams in the Night

A study-tour group of university students had arrived at a sister university campus in the interior of Sichuan province, People's

Republic of China. A dormitory on the edge of Chengdu University of Science and Technology would be home for the next several months. As we settled in our rooms I gazed down upon the teeming citizenry, bicycling on busy streets below, and stared at high-rise apartments facing us just beyond them. Friendly hosts quickly reduced getting-acquainted anxieties. They and the great food and fascinating sights lived up to our highest expectations.

One disturbing element—occurring at night—would intervene. Sounds, strange and unfamiliar, could easily awaken one the first few nights. And one of them we all recognized: a piercing scream or two. Our study host acknowledged my query about this as well as the eerie and bizarre feelings these cries conjured up. At least some of the screams, he thought, might have come from certain family members struggling with their own apprehensions and inner torments: the mentally ill. For most of us an initial encounter with a symptom such as this arouses discomfort, even fear.

The impact we felt echoes in both modern and ancient cultures. In China, even today the stigma affects the entire family and not only the person who is ill. Such families are thought to carry hereditary traits of moral failure; in addition, marrying off children and maintaining the family's status in the community becomes that much more difficult.[15]

Citizens in the country of the Gerasenes in New Testament times went a step further. A man shouting and out of control (demon possessed) evidently posed a threat to social order. Subsequently they had him shackled and kept under guard until Jesus came along to end the whole crisis situation (Luke 8:26-39). When the townspeople saw the former tomb-dwelling outsider "sitting at the feet of Jesus clothed and in his right mind . . . they were seized with great fear," and asked Jesus to leave them alone (vs. 35-37). Why were the Gerasenes afraid? I prefer to think they were in awe and overwhelmed at this point. What a bizarre happening! Would the visiting wonder-worker now begin somehow to blackmail them with Voodoo-like curses? What would happen next? So they would rather not linger under his thrall; best to try forgetting about "demons" completely.

A similar attitude hovers around us as well. Powerful stigma accompanies talk about mental illness, as if you (like Bill or Carol) or your parents must have done something terribly wrong. According to a publication of the U.S. Department of Health and Human Services, the American public has concluded that the two worst things that can happen to a person are leprosy and mental illness. Moreover, even ex-cons stand higher on the ladder of public acceptance than someone with a "mental problem."[16]

Research reveals that, on the average, television viewers can find at least one "mentally ill person" on their home screens every night of the year. Moreover, this rate—adding the available multiple cable stations—steadily increases. And in the recent past, shows such as the popular *M*A*S*H*, in its 251 episodes over eleven seasons, portrayed frequent psychiatric themes. Some have also concluded that psychiatric illness is the number one health-related problem in the soap opera world.[17]

Newspaper headlines print "Sex predator: mental illness discussed" or—upon describing details of a particularly outrageous crime—will take note of a suspect "with a history of mental problems." Most individuals suffering this way are not assaultive or violent; the minority who do become so actually make a minor contribution to the broad context of America's violent society.[18] But observers would seldom come to such a conclusion given crime reports (the "insanity" defense), Hollywood's movies (*One Flew Over the Cuckoo's Nest*), and common parlance such as "psycho."

Furthermore, these shy and unwashed neighbors will suffer a private contempt that drags upon any confidence and self-respect they may still have left. I asked a group home member (as I gave him a lift) why he preferred to cash his public assistance check at a locale more distant than ones closer at hand. "They say 'hello' to me there," he replied.

The citizens of Gerasene country had decided to shun their shouting, violence-prone neighbor. Our own neighbors struggling with less dramatic symptoms can produce embarrassment, distrust, and fear in current society. The result? Not only rejection; we also assign legions of them to jail or to the streets.

The Last Taboo

Screams in the night and threats of violence *are* unsettling. Anthropologist Mary Douglas connects such felt stresses to the boundaries cultures maintain between the sacred and the profane. Animals, objects, or persons perceived as "polluted" would qualify as unholy and restricted under a taboo or social ban. Complexities emerge when, for example, in the Middle East pigs simultaneously are held to be unclean by some and sacred by others. One's socially defined condition might also be linked with the supernatural dangers of formidable spirits.[19]

It all rings true for the Luke 8 story above: the possessed man has incredible powers; yet he raves out there in the hills with the swine. For both human and beast, their boundaries had remained until Jesus appeared and erased them. But time and geography have limited such displays of the "Son of the Most High God's" power (vs. 28). And the taboo of neighbors we consider dirty or threatening and label "psychopath" or "neurotic" remains very much alive.

A 1957 study of public attitudes toward persons living with mental illness uncovers a strong negative tendency. Understood as dangerous and unpredictable, they "laugh more than normal people and pay little attention to their personal appearance." Moreover, supposedly content with themselves, they "purposely avoid professional help." Their behavior was thought to have been the result of financial and social problems; in addition, cure for these "insane" individuals would remain out of reach.[20] Such blame and shame notions thankfully are slowly disappearing.

In "Mission in a Violent World," a sermon based upon Luke 8:26-39, a preacher places the context of Christian mission today in a similar world of destructive forces, one with screams in the night. He exhorts listeners to recognize their presence while at the same time offering the power of God in Jesus Christ to claim victory over them. He concludes with an additional claim: Christian mission creates a new community of God that notably *includes* those once despised and excluded. Perhaps this is why the Gerasene citizens asked Jesus to leave their country.[21]

In recent decades our own taboo subjects such as human sexuality and "death and dying" have crossed boundaries of neglect, embarrassment, and fear. Will mental illness follow? Many of us can look back and gasp in wonder at memories of the racial segregation in our country. Thankfully now we can begin to see the start of perhaps the last great inclusion in American life, namely, hospitality for more of those with mental handicaps. Will the Church help lead the way?

To summarize, I have begun with a picture of the presence of troubled and anxious perceptions ("dis-ease") within the ones who must cope with mental disorders; with the uninitiated in mind I have continued with a sketch of new "medicalized" treatment, and portrayed some current public attitudes about the subject. A part of the latter population warrants special attention. Hence I turn next to the environment of families living daily in its company.

Chapter 2

Family Impact

Occasionally, the mentally ill make headlines through random acts of violence; given our legal system's endorsement of "the right to be crazy," the miracle is that these incidents are not more frequent . . . the victims of the mentally ill are much more commonly their own families.

Rael Isaac and Virginia Armat
*Madness in the Streets:
How Society and the Law
Abandoned the Mentally Ill*

As she thinks about family chaos and the imprint of her son's gradual loss of himself in delusion and hallucinations, a mother reflects:

Did any of us see it coming? When did he first start changing? We kept trying to fix things. The quarrels, scenes, failures, and screaming continued, no matter what we did. Our love could not stop the inevitable push toward insanity. Now, twenty years later, it is even worse in some ways: a quiet withdrawal into nothingness . . .[1]

From remembering a series of false hopes, she reels toward despair. But an inner resolve affirms that family members will persevere and move beyond the defeats of madness for everyone trying to "fix things." Their question, "Whatever caused it, genes or environment?" goes begging. Deciding to establish a focus upon the needs of their family member, they will recognize his or her own burdens and the courage represented by the smallest gain.[1] Many other families across the continents trace this pattern.

The story will likely begin with the shock of having to make a diagnosis of family helplessness that could never have been imagined. Future run-ins with relapses from treatment failures will bump the sojourners along the way, and a backlash of unresolved grieving lingers on through the months and years. Family victims can include spouses, children, siblings, and grandparents, as well as extended family. Before their very eyes, they notice loved ones becoming strangers. Consider some common threads selected from family histories.

TUMULTS AND SHOUTING

Schizophrenia often afflicts people from postadolescence on into their twenties. Occurring just at the time young people leave home, episodes of unusual behavior can appear as an expected part of the hubbub involved in growing up—poor grooming, apathy, unusual eating and sleeping habits. Yet popular Australian media personality Anne Deveson saw more and would become both distressed and worried about her son Jonathan's behavior. She writes:

> Adolescence can be a time of extremes, from rebellious independence to agonizing vulnerability; a time to burst through into the adult world and find your own identity. In front of our eyes, his personality was slowly changing. I felt as if he were caught in a maze of terror, and I was on the outside struggling to free him but I could not find the way.[2]

Maggie always knew Ruth was different. There would be anger and hurt when Ruth's behavior embarrassed her daughter and her sisters, but the thought of mental illness was still alien to their world. When Maggie went away to college, for example, there was a day when Ruth called for her every fifteen minutes, around the clock. "That's my mother," she told her curious roommates and offered no further explanation. But finally, when Ruth was taken to a psychiatrist, even then Maggie was stunned; she had always thought her mother somewhat "crazy," but not *crazy.* "It was bizarre," she recalls, "but it explained so many questions about my whole life . . . liberating and horrible at the same time." The psychiatrist couldn't understand how the family had been living with what husband Art described to him. "You are not doing her a service," he concluded.[3]

Delusions about religious matters are quite common in cases of severe mental disturbance. Sometimes, for instance, a person is convinced of his or her eternal damnation, spending hours each day searching the Bible for forgiveness. A woman wrote to "Dear Abby":

> My husband is obsessed with sin and my supposed sins in particular. He is also overly concerned about being poor, to the point where he dragged out a piece of toast from the rubbish and insisted that we eat it. He counts the meatballs for the spaghetti, allowing only two per person, and he gets very upset when I want to add a few extra.[4]

Odd behavior such as this will confound both reason and remedy strategies. Continued for weeks and months on end, would-be supporters or helpers find themselves stressed to the point of exhaustion. "My grief was so raw," writes Anne Deveson, "that I often had a pain in my stomach . . . I felt like a fruit tree whose branches had been picked bare."[5]

Frightening episodes erupted when Jack and Lucille tried to deal with Tony, their recent college drop-out son. Having seen themselves as ordinary citizens in an ordinary household, it seemed now as if they had set up house in a minefield. The family usually had dinner together. Still, as Lucille recaptures one evening's explosion:

> Tony invariably seemed to be angry. Sometimes he just shouted loud, ugly words, sometimes he would throw things: bits of food, a spoon, his napkin. One time he sat down and Jack said: "How was your day, Tony?" Tony didn't answer; he just took his arm and swept everything—everything off the table onto the floor. Food, dishes, and cutlery were strewn every which way all over the kitchen. Jack and I (Lucille shakes her head) we both wept.[6]

At first these family rows remain private. Affected family members refuse to abandon hope for a way out and recovery of their loved one's old self. Another reason may involve a "life cannot really be like this" denial of the mess. Physical effects, however, are bound to creep into the picture.

The pastor's "couldn't care less" depression symptom (identified in the previous chapter) likely led to insomnia spells and to excessive worry and anger in his spouse. It is easy to imagine Jack and Lucille's marital strain, and the self-imposed guilt of a parental judgement: where did we go wrong? From the viewpoint of the sufferers themselves, the inner voices and ghostly visions of Bill, Jess, and Carol spawned fear and fatigue. People become drained; denial collapses in surrender to bitter admissions of helplessness. "What comes next?" they ask themselves.

Researchers at the University of Michigan found in 1990 that 40 percent of Americans seek help from clergy for their mental health needs. However, at the same time, the early 1990s also saw dozens of clergy confronted with malpractice lawsuits. Accustomed to feeling free to talk with parishioners about most of life's troubles, today's pastors are beginning to have second thoughts. Trying to guide people through seasons of melancholy, marital problems, and family upheavals has turned into a litigation minefield. Hence they are starting to assume more of a "gatekeeper" role and more often refer parishioners to professional counselors. Some will limit the number of times they will see someone on a one-on-one basis and ask secretaries to witness personal conversations. In an "anxious paralysis" over threatening lawsuits, and to avoid being held to the same standards as secular psychologists, a few will draw back in silence. Still another remarks how he has guided conversations with congregation members "away from changes in their lives, loss, death, marriage, family issues and acting-out children" to matters of God and faith. Colleagues will meet with the person, "listen to them, make conversation in terms of their faith, and pray with them."[7] *Listening* and *praying* catch my attention here. In other words, such a response leaps back over counselor and gatekeeper roles simply to *being present* amidst family struggles over mental illness and treatment issues. And this, I argue, helps most in the long run.

SHALOM *IN A BOTTLE?*

"Above all, some *peace*," family victims mutter to themselves, "no more prisoners to madness." Seeking out the minister or family doctor usually comes first. Provided the shame and guilt are not overly pronounced, maybe an old friend, former teacher, or "senior citizen" extended family member could provide a sympathetic ear. Victim lock-outs from the house as a last resort or, if fortunate enough, contact with a community mental health center might work. For some, it could mean simply dialing 911.

The Hebrew word for "peace" (*shalom*) occurs some 250 times in the Bible and has a variety of usages. Besides the courteous greeting (Gen. 43:23) and the social meaning of good relationships between peoples or nations (Judg. 4:17), *shalom* defines tranquility and contentment (Psalm 119:165). There are also connotations of the Creator's sustenance (Psalms 4:8), and even health and its restoration (Gen. 15:15; Ex. 18:7; Josh. 10:21; I Kings 22:17). In the New Testament, the Greek word (*eirene*) makes a further distinction of the peace resulting from the mediation of Jesus Christ for the salvation of humankind (Rom. 5:1; Eph. 2:14-17).[8]

Indeed, all of the meanings above are desirable outcomes. Yet one of them stands out as the key to the second step of respite beyond the first intervention: tranquility. Little wonder that the medications prescribed in psychiatric care (see Chapter 1) are nicknamed "tranquilizers." These elixirs can quell anger; they calm people down enough to accept the refuge of a quiet hospital ward and clean bed in place of street jungles. For family members the quiet and calm face of brother, sister, child, or parent as opposed to the former scowl or tic provides a deep relief; finally, no more agitation and pacing! Furthermore, possibilities always seem to lie just over the horizon for healing words of forgiveness and hopes for a fresh start.

Tony decided he would like to go back to school. He enrolled again and—to the delight of his parents—reported regularly to Dr. Reid for talk therapy in the process. Besides, he was taking his prescribed "meds" on schedule. At last, Jack and Lucille rejoiced, the nightmare was behind them. But wait. Tony, loving his courses, doing well and flushed with mounting success, became certain he was not really sick after all. He stopped seeing Dr. Reid and tossed the medication bottles in the wastebasket.

The resultant deterioration was swift and dramatic. Because he was surly and irritable once more, Tony's campus friends began backing off. The old shouts of hostility doused optimism at home; sadness and frustration took over. "Back to square one," concluded Jack and Lucille.[9]

Jonathan Deveson also tried to make it on his own. He took up with several old friends from high school, but no one would live with him more than a few days. Too chaotic, they said. Sometimes people cheated him and his mother would come to the rescue. Without her continued interventions for one thing or another, like a homing pigeon he would return (usually in the middle of the night) to the household. A major reason for the slide was that once more Jonathan had stopped taking his medication. Anne explains:

> At this stage the only way to get Jonathan back onto medication would have been to enforce it. But he was not psychotic enough to be involuntarily committed, and this has been a major flaw in mental health legislation—or its administration—around the world. You watch someone you love becoming psychotic, but you can do nothing until they are so ill that they are judged to be a danger to themselves or others. I used to wonder how society would react if we took the same approach with a physical illness. If someone had an infected leg, for instance, what would happen if we made them wait until it were gangrenous before giving any medical help?[10]

Family members are caught between two peacemaker intervention opposites: on the one hand, the physical intervention is intended to rescue. On the other hand, rescue can also mean withdrawing all support in favor of creating self-reliance and independence. *Shalom* from a bottle remains tantalizing but elusive.

GRIEF WORK

Scholarly discussion of the familiar opening sentences of the Bible (Gen. 1:1-2:4a) locates their poetic power in the worship of

God at the Jerusalem temple. Praise of the Lord as Creator is paramount. The worship sentences (liturgy) celebrate new life; the dark, formless empty chaos has been turned into a world of divine order and purpose. The worshipping community in turn participates in the victory over the forces of disorder.[11] When earthquakes, floods, tornados, and brush fires persist, however, worshippers can recognize that the conquest still appears limited and uncertain.

The community represented by Anne Deveson, Maggie, and Tony's parents quickly learns caution about triumph in terms of personal events. Observers will eventually hear about one factor continuing to unite each of their stories: chaos. Unpredictability, uncontrolled temper, senseless speech, and bizarre acts can once more define "dark, formless, and empty" puzzles. Although our culture accepts the language of people "going crazy" or "insane," or "losing their minds," they know realities of *mental disorder.*

A second unifying sphere shaping this community will involve a sense of loss. The affected person's "old self" may disappear during acute episodes or for longer periods of time. Personality changes, and not for the better. Furthermore, amidst their anger and frustration, those who want to help lose confidence in themselves and how to apply what they have learned from prior life events in situations such as these. Advice from others also falters in the melee. It all adds up, and grieving enters life.

Loss by death is normally associated with grieving. A person suffers bereavement (to be "cut off" or "torn up"), for example, from the sudden death of a loved one; when it happens as a result of violence, the happening can make people feel as if an outside force has taken violent, destructive action against them. The more anticipated loss—after lengthy illness, for instance—can nevertheless create "torn up" emotions of having been deprived against one's will.

Besides being a reaction to loss, grief also refers to a person's response to bereavement; beyond the "I cannot believe it!" anguish loom distress and heartbreak. The term "mourning" also comes to mind. It suggests the longer process of coping with loss in a given community or society.[12] Societal scripts are provided for grievers and community sympathy is offered according to accepted norms for armed services-related deaths, for example, or for accidents on the road, or at the nursing home. Not all loss, however, is so visible, or makes the newspapers to be sanctioned by society. Suicide, AIDS deaths, and death occurring during a crime illustrate this. Abortion sadness and grieving linked with mental incompetence are others. This is "disenfranchised grief" and complicates our understanding of bereavement.[13]

The unique grief felt by family members mentioned here earlier remains a total mystery to so many of our neighbors; such loss is not even recognized on a list of the hidden and unrecognized grieving prepared by professional students of the subject. Theorists among them have proposed a "grief work" model to help us understand better the effects of loss—the basic source of grieving—in our everyday lives.[14]

The model has three facets. The first task involves accepting the reality of the loss. With the death of a loved one, this can mean a painful but deliberate move from saying, "he or she *is* a talented . . ." to "he or she *was* a talented . . ." With severe mental disorders the "is" nevertheless remains while both the talent and personality seem to have died. Such a duality is unique and the pain involved becomes difficult even to talk about with others, making the acceptance of loss that much more difficult. Further, hope survives and grasps at cure: diet? different medications? another physician? Jonathan Deveson even went to India in search of alternative treatment. How about religion? One waits . . . and dreams.

Meanwhile, the chaos continues in one pattern or another. It arises when those marvelous tranquilizing medications produce unpleasant side effects in some individuals. Probably as a result of their dopamine-restricting functions, side effects include head, neck, and body twistings; facial tics and grimaces can make onlookers frown back. Muscles can stiffen and eyes will roll. It's enough to make a healthy loved one weep. Thank goodness, they learn, such symptoms are usually temporary; others, however, may persist. Prominent are unwanted weight gain plus feelings of apathy and drowsiness. At the opposite end of this scale, tremors and a feeling of restlessness make an affected individual feel compelled to be constantly on the move. Thus, people on medication need to be monitored carefully.[15]

The second "grief work" undertaking means working through the pain of loss. This requires a discipline of avoiding comfort through nonprescription (or prescription) drugs and self-medication through use of alcohol. Reaching out to others for social support may help in moving through bereavement; recalling happy events and perhaps even the use of humor can heal as well. But in the case of someone suffering from severe mental disorder the privation becomes impossible to relegate to past—and sometimes romanticized—life events. The expressionless, silent, and sober visage of your kin stares right back at you. Yet the pain comes also from unforseen realities. The distressing condition known as tardive dyskinesia will occasionally manifest itself, especially among the elderly. This technical term identifies involuntary movements of the face and tongue; once seen it is seldom forgotten. Science as yet understands little about this problem. A tranquilizer regimen seems to cause it in some cases, yet sometimes it occurs apart from medication treatments. What a sad choice remains—to abandon sufferers to the horrors of unrelieved psychosis or to keep on with drugs and hope for the best? Thus the hope of "getting on with your life," or working through by "moving forward" must stay on hold a bit longer.

The third function of the model implies making an adjustment to a changed environment in which the deceased is missing. This could mean rearranging the furniture, travel, or reorganizing family rituals. Yet for family members like Anne, Art, and Maggie, it could mean simply trying to counter the changing habits, new slovenliness, foul language, or off-hours of the parent, child, spouse, or sibling.[16]

Severe mental disorders produce shock, dismay, and confusion within a family circle. Some abdicate from care attempts and lock their doors or flee. Others will continue to vie with crisis episodes and stay alive despite the ambiguity and self-destructiveness of it all. As a result spouses and parents, children, siblings, and sometimes extended family members continue to sorrow in defeat. In wrestling with loss these victims must also adapt to extended grief work.

Dealing with one's own depression may become important. Resentment surfaces and one mutters, "Why did this happen to us? Others get by just fine!" or, "It's just not fair, this whole sorry business!" This mood arises in part because of an all-or-nothing thinking: "My relative has no life because he or she has schizophrenia . . . there is nothing going for that person."[17] In fact, however, he or she nevertheless *has* a life and is capable of feelings and accomplishments. The cognitive distortion on the caregiver's part cites a grain of truth that is then exaggerated to a maladaptive degree. Self-defeating beliefs such as "My relative *shouldn't* give me such a hard time" could adapt instead to an alternative line for dealing with depression: "I would prefer it if my relative didn't give me such a hard time. What can I do to change the problem?" Or, furthermore, instead of "It's unfair that I have to suffer like this when I don't deserve it," try "Nobody likes to suffer. Is there something I can do to improve this situation?"[18]

"Time marches on," as early media newsreels announced. As its progress stretches over months and years, whatever it is that brings about mental disorder in an individual's brain and personality can also create new challenges in the family circle. "Cure" conversations are gradually silenced and repentance emerges. By this familiar biblical term (Mark 1:14-15), I mean "to think again," to turn around and change one's mind. It underscores a dynamic transition from one state to another. The conversion may mean a break with past habits and behavior; it can also point to the future, to revised attitudes and new pathways in life.[19]

Chapter 3

From Madhouse to Mad House

At some point, it becomes clear that family members need to continue on with their individual lives and begin to think of supporting their ill loved one over the long run. This is when coping begins to take the place of grieving.

LeRoy Spaniol and Anthony M. Zipple
Psychological and Social Aspects of Psychiatric Disability

Anne Deveson could begin working through the painful loss of her son by telling others about it in her gripping story. Tony's parents, Jack and Lucille, and Maggie—Ruth's daughter—bravely adjusted to and compromised with bizarre and undreamed-of family environments. As far as actually *accepting* the realities of serious mental illness, however, things were different. When hints of recovery and even hopes for rehabilitation began to dawn, they convinced themselves of light at their tunnel's end. But a sudden relapse collapsed the fragile structure. Defeat and grief work's journey through the pain resumed. Challenges discussed in Chapter 1—breakdowns in the sufferer, elusive symptoms, and the threat of stigma—return to the pilgrim pathways.

For family members the burdens will sometimes recall laments such as David's:

Save me, O God, for the waters have come up to my neck.
I sink in deep mire, where there is no foothold;
I have come to deep waters, and the flood sweeps over me.
I am weary with crying; my throat is parched.
My eyes grow dim with waiting for my God. (Psalm 69:1-3)

THE WAITING FAMILY

Heir to a fortune, the hard-working farmer could put up with it no longer. His younger brother, the "prodigal son" of a famous parable (Luke 15:11-32) had broken family rules and boundaries again and taken off to live it up abroad. And now, upon the wastrel's profligacy and eventual exhaustion, he was supposed to join a happy *celebration* of the prodigal's homecoming? So—bitterly protesting— the older brother refuses the parental invitation, citing his own loyalty and clean living in contrast to the rascal's public disgrace (vs. 25-32).

A "classic manipulation," he fumed, that "half-grown-up, irresponsible kid" was back; yet not only was his foolishness overlooked, the failures were not even penalized. Still, a festive holiday mood banished the gloom, or did it? The father soon discovered an elder sibling's resentment and voiced a plea to counter it. "But we had to celebrate and rejoice because this brother of yours was dead and has come to life; he was lost and has been found (vs. 32). Rembrandt's masterpiece displays the kneeling son's pleading humiliation. The artist focuses light upon the father's compassionate face and forgiving hands. Yet we can almost hear the drumbeat of the brother's resentment as he stares off in the distance.

How often have churchgoers listened to Luke's parable in sermons that ignore the dependable brother's slow burn and righteous indignation? Likely his protest was a speech he had rehearsed for months. Normally, it seems we in the pews have been tuned to the joyous surprises of forgiveness and reconciliation from the "waiting father."[1]

Earlier in Luke, a woman named Martha had been trying to prepare a proper welcome for a famous visitor to her home. But inside she was becoming rather vexed. Instead of helping out when she was verging on dismay because of kitchen tasks, her sister Mary just sat there—listening to Jesus (Luke 10:38-42). In a sketch of this episode, Rembrandt shows Jesus and Mary in pleasant table conversation; Martha, in contrast, is depicted simply as a shadowy blob hunched at the fireplace nearby. Again, it seems like strange justice here when once more the boundary breaker's behavior has involved the "better part" in the Master's appraisal (vs. 42).[2]

It often happens that way in families distracted by serious mental illness. To affected brothers and sisters sometimes parents seem endlessly preoccupied with an irresponsible sibling. They themselves, it seems, are taken for granted. Moreover, parents appear never to have mustered the courage to say "no" in the face of these manipulators, who always angle for a break and never have to pay the price for rebellion and destructive (substance abuse) behaviors.

In her book, *Mad House*, Clea Simon recalls how it was to grow up in the shadow of mentally ill siblings:

> Many of us have found ourselves doubly wounded; first by our family experience and then by a lack of comprehension—in ourselves as well as others—as to why we are needy, hurt, angry, disconnected. As "healthy" siblings we have wondered if our experience even counts; after all, we are not suffering the tragic and inexplicable illnesses of our brothers and sisters. But we, too, have come through tragedies, no matter if the degree and details differ, and we have all been changed by them.[3]

For most of us it takes time to accept behavior that defies our sense of basic right and wrong. Thielicke's "waiting father" contradicts the smug and satisfying "I told you so" of an expected revenge. Forgiveness and compassion had replaced getting even. He had wiped the slate clean; a new start became the top priority. And while sympathizing with Martha, we have to admit the basic rightness of the "better part" her Guest was sharing with Mary.

It often works out like this for parents coping with long-term mental illness. You forgive the 3:00 a.m. door-rattling sleep disturbances while anticipating a normal night's rest tomorrow. You relent and provide yet another ride to the psychiatrist's office (just this once, lest you become a prodigal's "enabler"). You bite your nails and give in again because of a dream that by next week or next month the nightmare will cease; we will have turned the corner toward the blessings of peace and normality.

Society's response can remain tentative until troubled ones are sufficiently mentally ill; for instance, we seek to learn if a dangerous act—such as attacking a bus driver with a cane while muttering "assassination"—has come about as yet. Such behavior could lead to hospital commitment. Yet, as a consequence, treatment then becomes *criminalized*. Compassion counts for nothing. Little wonder people have such a hard time admitting impulsive indiscretions, spending money they shouldn't have, and becoming sexually involved with people they shouldn't. Punitive and jail care approaches are not the answer.[4]

Anne, college dropout daughter of Shirley and Neal Matthews, could not hold a job longer than a few weeks. Eventually the other members of Anne's family found themselves chasing helter skelter to mental agencies, hospitals, and to law enforcement centers. The family became driven with these affairs, "checking up on Anne." Life began to take on a splintered, fragmented, and desperate character. Worries could consume the day. Separation would be a good idea for everyone, they concluded, and helped Anne into her own apartment.

She decorated it nicely and visits were exchanged on an arrangement that seemed at first an answer to a prayer. But soon it was apparent that while living apart from her siblings and parents Anne became isolated socially. Moreover, when meals were shared, they noted, she was clearly delusional, certain her neighbors were poisoning her food. Before long Anne returned home. As Shirley recalled the outcome:

> Our daughter lived in our house, and it was as though she were a ghost. . . . We knew that she slipped down to the kitchen to eat. I would put things out for her, and I wrote little notes on the refrigerator trying to tempt her to eat something that I had made especially for her.[5]

Finally, Neal warned his daughter about such behavior and challenged her to "take some responsibility" for her own life.

Early the next morning, Anne, fully dressed, left the house. Expecting her to return before dark, Shirley and Neal sat in the kitchen, drinking tea and checking the time; but no Anne, either on the phone or at the door. Two months went by until they got a call from a detective in a neighboring state. Here was their Anne, in the police station, calling for help in tracking down members of the KGB.

Yet when the social worker called to the scene concluded that her client intended harm neither to herself nor others, and that she was clean, well-fed, and had shelter, she told Anne Matthews she was free to leave. But Anne never made it back to the shelter. Other than a rumor of a possible sighting in Seattle, this would be the last specific word Neal and Shirley Matthews would hear of the whereabouts of their daughter. Their note to her at the city Metro Crisis line reads:

> We realize you have a right to do what you wish to do, but we want you to know we miss you and would like you to come home. Your Dad and Mom, and sisters still love you.[6]

Muddled family denials breed grief, anxieties, and guilt. Add the continual failures of efforts to save and the first shockwave of our mental illness depiction surfaces: helplessness.

SURFING THE SYSTEM

Despair shadows helplessness. Is it even a loss of hope that stirs King David's cry of distress?

> How long, O Lord? Will you forget me forever?
> How long will you hide your face from me?
> How long must I bear pain in my soul, and have sorrow in my heart all day long?
> How long shall my enemy be exalted over me? (Psalm 13:1-2)

Family members trying to cope with the behavior of a loved one with serious mental illness in their midst will gradually learn how in sadness. Not everything in life qualifies as positive and romantic; situations will not always submit to control or management. Furthermore, they realize that polite and civil exchanges at mealtime, for example, should be treasured and never taken for granted.

Yet, like ancient Judah at the fall of Jerusalem, they can also sense God's presence in exile (Psalm 137:1-6) and prepare for the second shockwave, namely, a chronic, long-term prospect. One mother reflects:

> There are things we can do, however, and one of these is to remain loyal for the long haul. The place in our hearts is as big as ever, though we often do not know what to say or do. But we have not abandoned you, beloved, and we never will.[7]

Often the media today reminds us about advances in science and medicine. Research and treatment work the now-familiar wonders of heart surgery, liver transplants, and more effective drugs in the battle against AIDS. I join the applause. Moreover, given a political will tied to technological advances, we assume similar benefits will continue to roll in. Some may even dream about advances in life expectancy figures to who knows where? After all, "they (scientists) are even cloning sheep."

Have we forgotten something amidst such triumphs of progress? An unstated disclaimer may stem from an attitude toward the body; while the bodies of others actually weaken and grow older, we ourselves do not. Hence, our society's unspoken resolve to depend upon scientists, new treatments, and technologies to fend off physical threats lingers on. A flight from mortality looms large in our society. Ads for instant cures—plus hints of total wellness—become an ideology's watchwords, implying that life need not be marred by excess pain or disability. We want to take charge, fix things, and control matters.

But "mental illness" families have to wait months and even years for the slightest signs of cure and wholeness in an affected one's life. *Vulnerability* begins to dawn in their consciousness; folks learn that *being perfect* is a bit out of reach as well. Sometimes dreams are not even partly fulfilled. Still, human impotence is not a curse; it is a "gift which frees us from having to be like God!"[8] Despite isolation and defeats, siblings such as Clea and parents such as Anne's can refuse to give up and adapt instead. This involves first-hand experience with the professional mental illness caregiving system.

By "system" I mean the caregiving network supported by medical, legal, and social work professionals. Like TV channel-switching "surfers," caregiving families will eventually resort to bouncing around their local venues. In her handbook, *When Someone You Love Has a Mental Illness*, Rebecca Woolis distinguishes various players on a community team.[9] They include:

1. *Psychiatrist*—an MD specialist qualified to prescribe medication.
2. *Psychologist*—with six to eight years of postgraduate training (often including a PhD), these individuals are prepared to consult and to administer psychological testing.

3. *Social Worker*—normally holding a master's degree in social work, these team players will consult about available housing, job training opportunities and so forth.
4. *Others*—including psychiatric nurses (RNs) plus occupational and recreational therapists.

In treating different illnesses, a doctor (MD) oversees the overall course of treatment. This does not often happen in cases of mental disorders since the doctor is unable or unwilling to follow the illness course once the patient has left the hospital. Thus our fifth team member, the *case manager*, comes into play. These professionals (social work, counseling, or psychology) help with transitions involving vocational and practical needs.[10] They assist clients in applying for financial benefits including Social Security aid such as Supplemental Security Income (SSI) and disability insurance.

With the advent of psychotropic medication, during the 1960s the majority of chronically ill patients were discharged from the state hospitals for continued treatment in the community. In 1963, President Kennedy's administration passed the Community Mental Health Centers Act. Consequently, about 800 geographically defined zones were outlined in each agency-arranged "catchment area." Centers were created (community mental health centers, CMHCs) for the purpose of helping discharged psychiatric patients cope more effectively outside the hospital. They began to provide a wide range of services, including evaluations, case management, day treatment programs, occupational therapy, referrals, and others. Many are today also affiliated with community residences, and transportation and educational programs.[11]

With this sketch of the caregiving system organization in mind, let us turn to the dynamics of its operation in the fictional case of eighteen-year-old Bill and his parents. Alcohol and drug abuse combined with teenage recklessness has resulted in a couple of DWI (driving while intoxicated) brushes with the law. Worse still, night-long absences from home plus stomping rages when confronted with them hinted at something desperately amiss. (Could it *be*? Mental disorder in *our* family?)

At the time of crisis, the hospital emergency room and psychiatric ward provided help, giving respite to, in this case, anxious parents and a vulnerable, sick youth. The immediate goal was to stabilize the erratic behavior arising from his symptoms of delusion and hallucination. But legal requirements (voluntary vs. involuntary commitment) imposed an urgent seventy-two-hour time frame in which it must be determined if Bill were "a danger to himself or others." By what procedure? As a result, long-range goals of well-being and health were sometimes cut short by ill-timed releases and by the patient's own subsequent alcohol and street drug interference with the prescribed medical regimen. The stage was set for rehospitalization and a downward spiral toward chronic illness.

Assuming an eventual adequate stabilization time frame, the second set of surroundings for the family was the "recovering arena." This inched beyond crisis dynamics to a suspenseful search for just the right living arrangement, medication, or employment opportunity to put Bill back on his feet. Caregivers included social workers, psychologists, congregate care center workers, and social clubs sponsored by the mental health center. Helping actions such as counseling, as well as providing security for the client and assistance in discovering relevant social networks (support groups) combined to ensure respite and a measure of relief. The family church, aloof and silent, seemed irrelevant to treatment at the time.

The third caregiving context, a "plateau" or long-term situation, marked the beginning of meaningful pastoral care. Over the months as Bill's stubborn symptoms of blunted affect (apathy), poverty of speech, and social withdrawal lingered on, pastors first helped by listening to the story, so far as family members could tell it. When asked, one pastor gave effective respite help as a protective payee to receive subsistence checks in the absence of the parents. Yet it was reactive help, never a proactive initiative. Meanwhile, the emotional burdens of anxiety, resentment, grief, and depression—however hidden and unexpressed—took their toll upon both parent and sibling.

The chaos surrounding the demands created by the illness of their loved one was compounded by the bureaucratic labyrinth—doctors who refused to communicate with parents, insufficiently funded programs, and the stance of our problem-solving culture I mentioned earlier. We isolate the problem as though it were a traffic tie-up and take steps to "solve" it. Solutions are assumed. Most of the time we enter hospitals and take medications as an answer and cure. But in a continued bout with mental illness participants begin to recognize something different. *Years* go by and answers seem to elude doctors and everyone else.

ABSORBED

Illness, argues Arthur Kleinman, always carries social as well as personal meanings.[12] Signs of helplessness and chronicity, despite days of hope following intervals of defeat, can jolt us from boundaries of ordinary reality. Each family will come to terms with the results in its particular environment. The illness experience need not always bring defeat. Even if disappointment often results—especially in stories of serious mental illness—the "adventure" can also become an element for growth, a point of departure for something deeper and better in life. New meanings are created. One of them concerns the healing potentials for shaping treatment alliances of the untrained parent, spouse, and sibling with the professional caregiver working in the system.

Two Visions of Health

Illness definitions should be shared and negotiated. In the case of our topic, families of the long-term mentally ill will likely have views of health and well-being different from those held by mental health professionals. Their image often stresses coping responses over a lifetime of their own caregiving or procured through social services agencies.

In contrast, mental health professionals hold an image placing less emphasis upon ongoing family involvement than upon separation and autonomy. Professionals believe this latter view corresponds to psychologically based treatment goals. Yet with case overloads and noncooperation (lack of medication compliance, for instance) from clients, trained caregivers suffer treatment reverses and disappointments similar to family setbacks. They, too, will wait for breakthroughs to success, however modest. Their goal becomes family therapy and cure; families, in contrast, long for more immediate help and support. They need information and assistance in

managing symptoms, help in accessing system resources, and discussion of long-range treatment plans.[13] Tensions between these
two dreams of health will arise when either the professional feels
undervalued or the family feels left out of the treatment process. But
if clinicians hear families' insights on patient behavior and families
learn about treatment intentions, clarifications can establish goals
both system and family members can mutually affirm.

Bill began to notice a change in his parents' activities. His mother,
in particular, reached out to other folks floundering in similar ways.
She was on the phone a lot, browsed for new books on mental
illness, and doubled her connections with the region's Alliance for
the Mentally Ill group. She also encouraged her mate to join in
sharing experiences and offering advice. Even Bill could sense that
they were no longer surfing but were actually immersed in the
caregiving system.

The social factors of working for better treatment or cures will
include use of three seldom-examined terms. The first, *disease*, is
the problem from the practitioner's perspective. It embraces biological terminology and a biomedical response strategy. *Sickness*, the
next word, calls attention to macrosocial economic and political
forces by connecting, for example, the incidence of tuberculosis to
poverty. *Illness* testifies to the human experience of symptoms of
disease and suffering, and to how the wider social network (family
in this case) perceives, lives with, and responds to them.[14] Symptoms and disability create illness problems. We may suffer loss of
hope for cure and become demoralized; we may grieve over lost
health, fear becoming an invalid, or feel shamed. Meanings com-
municated over the course of long-term serious mental illness can
both amplify and dampen such symptoms. Any attempts to stabilize
conditions, events, and human links in reacting to them will continue to demand creative efforts from caregivers.

Looking Ahead

The biblical case of Job presents a famous "illness problem."
Upon witnessing their friend's social and physical losses, Eliphaz,
Bildad, and Zophar try to communicate a caring response (Job
4:1-31:40). Their efforts wilt in the face of the victim's protest of

personal integrity: "Let me be weighed in a just balance, and let God know my integrity!" (Job 31:6).

Eventually, if nothing seems to work in recovery efforts, the question will surface: "What did we do to deserve the catastrophes of schizophrenia in our lives?" Sometimes, then, reality dictates acceptance of a long-term, gravely disabling and handicapping condition. But at the same time we can also learn from Job that while life is not always "fair," we can nevertheless adapt to and reach beyond heartbreak and bafflement as God's own servant did (Job 42:1-6). A thoughtful reflection upon the two previous visions of health could help put to use practical applications. Consider how a licensed counselor and director of a family support program (who, furthermore, has spent years of service working with people with mental illness) organizes them.[15] Teamwork to divide responsibility for treatment, she maintains, is basic.

The ill relative:

> Cooperates with system team members; attempts more personal behavior responsibility.

The family:

1. Offers love by ongoing supportive contacts with, for example, residential treatment centers of group homes.
2. Cooperates in treatment.
3. Educates its members about the illness and the system.

The doctors:

1. Provide a long-term therapeutic relationship, including an updated overview and prognosis.
2. Prescribe and monitor medication, educate about effects and side effects.

The case manager:

1. Assists the ill person with essential needs and stability in community social relationships.

2. Makes referrals to various treatment programs and attempts treatment continuity.
3. Provides crisis intervention as feasible.

The treatment-program staff provides:

1. Ongoing support activities, treatment plans, and therapeutic relationships.
2. Education, training, and counseling in interpersonal skills and vocational goals.
3. Documentation of the course of treatment.

The power of God, says St. Paul (1 Cor. 1:18-25), is revealed in weakness and supremely in the weakness of Jesus Christ. The paradox that true power may arise from apparent failure is revealed in the shameful death of an itinerant rabbi at the hands of a ruthless empire.

Parents such as ourselves behold failure in the lives of our children who remain dependent as adults with no employment, profession, or families of their own (in contrast to siblings). Parents see them linger on between the world of a child and the responsibilities of an adult. Before long parents must consider their future absence, and plan their wills accordingly. The author of a book outlining potential pastoral response to the suffering tied to tragic death has titled it, *When Faith Is Tested.* The art of pastoral follow-up, he argues, is critical and too easily forgotten in the "difficult weeks and months" following a grievous loss.[16] But the art will also apply to the periodic struggles of parents and other family members persevering through the years. These chronic illness interims suggest a title variation to Zurheide's text: "When Faith Is Tested . . . and Tested Again."

Yet, as their caregiving and life journey unfolds, these are the ones most apt to be taken aback in wonder at the Master's announcement that "whoever gives even a cup of water to one of these little ones . . . truly, I tell you, none of these will lose their reward" (Matt. 10:42) and "But many who are first will be last, and the last will be first" (Mark 10:31).

Where is the Church, the people of God, in these affairs? Where are its leaders and clergy? Are there any teamwork prospects out there? Let me investigate blessings and possibilities.

Chapter 4

Negotiating Contact

Coping depends upon those efforts persons make to master conditions of threat, harm, or challenge when the usual strategies are insufficient. Good copers are not destroyed by tragedy—they see it as a challenge to find solutions.

Victoria Secunda
When Madness Comes Home

The presence of the pastor provides another person to share the load. When a joy is shared by another, it is multiplied by two; when the sadness is shared, it is divided by two. Pastors do not perform magic, but they provide community for that other person. Similarly, they represent the presence of the living Christ.

Wayne E. Oates
Luck: A Secular Faith

Shock, denial, anger, and despair infiltrate the emotions of family caregivers and spread a virus of alienation. Most often the burden is concealed from others by internal family dynamics. In this chapter, I explore possibilities for outsiders to recognize these circles of pain with signs of public support.

On a recent sojourn in South Africa, I gave a series of lectures at Umphumulo Lutheran Seminary. My wife and I relied on the hospitality of staff members before eventually occupying a small guest cottage just off campus. We were pleased not to burden our busy hosts any further; besides, we would contribute more by becoming a little independent. It went well for a time; countryside walks, library browsing, and sharing meals at the student dining hall soon made us feel at home.

All at once, however, the matter of laundry came up. Coin-operated laundromats were left far behind in Durban. Alice managed the washing all right, but there was no clothesline. So we did our best and hung garments out to dry around windows and on the porch. Beyond them stretched a dramatic view of deep valleys with small farms dotting the forested hillsides.

Answering a knock on the door, I greeted a tall African man whom I had noticed sitting out on the porch of a cabin nearby, appreciating the same view. The language barrier surfaced but presented no problem. Smiling, and with a collapsible clothing rack in his hands, he offered us just what we needed.

Toward dusk on the day following, electrical power failed in the cottage and we found ourselves without flashlights or lanterns amidst another minicrisis. Again, with a soft knock our neighbor stood at the door. This time he furnished candles, holders, and matches. Later we learned that our benefactor lived alone and served as a campus handyman. To us he had become something more—a friendly neighbor and caregiver as well.

His reaching out touched our stay at Umphumulo in several ways. First, he recognized our presence as strangers who might have particular needs. Second, by overcoming perhaps a bit of hesitation ("Surely," he might have thought, "the principal will care for them"), he took the initiative to contact us. Last, the African neighbor's humble offerings extended tangible help; his contact had involved perception, initiative, and service. It lingers in memory.

Pastors and congregations can also find ways to support isolated families coping with long-lasting mental illness. But the effort will require education, determination, and persistence. And likely it will tax any caretaker's patience.

WHY WE HESITATE

I can understand why so many church people avoid even the topic of mental illness. Other ministries—youth, for example—cry out for attention. Besides, a steady flow of media reports can shape public inclinations to steer clear: a newspaper account of brutal murders reveals, for instance, the accused being found by doctors to have "a personality disorder with schizoid and paranoid features, delusions and hallucinations." No wonder readers assign the fallout to the police, courts, and hospitals. In cases where individuals have not been treated, I agree. Furthermore, drug and alcohol abuse plus noncompliance with medications can increase violent episodes.[1]

Yet, at the same time, many more nonviolent persons who faithfully comply with medication regimens stay with anxious relatives or in boarding homes where some act out Thoreau's "lives of quiet desperation." These often shy and modest individuals, along with their caregivers, represent today a silent parallel to the man in St. Paul's vision who pleaded, "Come over to Macedonia and help us" (Acts 16:9). To illustrate, consider the following.

A mother of teenagers, on medication for depression, discovers that her kids call her "crazy" to their friends. At home, her husband uses the word "psychopath" in discussing the treatment plan. Meanwhile, her depression deepens. Despite the family's church membership, rarely will a minister or parishioners even learn of her desperation, much less sympathize or minister.

Widowed at age thirty-nine, and the mother of two, another woman praises the pastor (who continued to call on them after her husband's funeral) and friends from church who knocked on the door like the African handyman did in our case. "They were there for us," she exclaims, "just when we needed them most." Crisis calls become publicly acknowledged blessings. But less urgent or public are those less frequent "chronic" visits to secluded and gravely troubled people. The "shut-ins" can become "shut-outs."

Yet often in cases of avoidance, it is important to stress how chronic sufferers and their families themselves are also to blame. They turn away from others in embarrassment and shame. When one mother shared an account of her son's disturbance, a pastor reported to me that she closed the conversation with, "Let's keep it quiet." Another parent explained, "At one point, my son closed himself up in his room for eighteen months. I left food for him and would try to peep into his window to see if he was all right."[2] Likely she kept thinking that if the family could endure just a little longer, a new medication or treatment procedure would come along and remove a nightmare best forgotten. The achievements of other "successful" families added up to humiliation and defeat for her own. Despair and apathy spawn social withdrawal.

Adding to it are well-meaning Christians who from ignorance communicate a message that mental disturbances are a result of sin or demon possession. Moreover, by believing the cause is simply poor parenting or abuse, they merely aggravate the pain.

Yet in contacts with people who have experienced the anguish—and through other learning initiatives—observers can learn to suspend such felt meanings. They will perceive prejudice and, through God's mercies, enable at least in part what Bible writers call redemption from such living hells (see, for instance, Exod. 21:30, Psalm 130:7, 1 Cor. 1:30).

A WORD IN SEASON

Should an acquaintance who happened to be a psychiatrist knock on the door or call for an appointment, likely most of us would be taken aback. "Why?" we would think, "What's the matter? What's wrong?" But if a pastor called (after assuring us that he or she was not bearing bad news), it would be different. Suspicions aside, a welcome chance for conversation about faith apart from business and job would have appeared instead.

Such an open access represents a unique professional advantage, one that can rank as both a pastoral duty and privilege. Only a couple of decades ago a pastor coming to call might expect to find someone home to welcome an unexpected guest. Yet today's pace usually requires taking the initiative for a meeting. Most families absorbed in coping with a loved one who is ill will drift to the margins of congregational life. Still, they long for some outside connections apart from routine contacts with mental health professionals or other families in the same circumstance. At this point clergy and members of congregations are ideally poised for ministry and support.

At the same time, however, the contact persons must not fail to try to become more aware of the often unusual coping skills represented in some of these families. For example, they gain expertise—worthy of health professional attention—in telling the difference between behaviors that are volitional and those that are caused by the illness itself.

Particularly when families themselves decide to act in response to mental disorders, creative ideas for their own survival will emerge. Observers have noted the most successful kinfolk copers are those who have at least one of three characteristics. The first targets secrecy: unpleasantness and sorrow notwithstanding, reliable information about the illness will be shared. Children are not kept in the dark. The second trait encourages well children's outside roles. These are not merely for escape, but are actively endorsed by parents who tell their offspring to strive for independence. The final trademark of good family coping makes clear (in the case of siblings) that responsibility for the ill person belongs to adults.[3] Any of these characteristics may open doors for meaningful conversation.

The Rivers family had long been active in First Church but in recent years problems had arisen with their son Randy. Rumors of drugs, school drop-outs, brushes with the law—driving while intoxicated and two wrecked cars—circled routinely. Hospital stays (even psychiatric!) completed the package.

Pastor Perry had called on Randy in the psych ward, to be sure, but got the impression from both the medics and the Rivers themselves that this outcome—being the last straw—had to be the prelude to Act I of the drama Rehabilitation. Months passed and no further word; there were no Rivers (siblings or parents) around church, either. Perry felt uneasy about it and began to wonder about checking back with them. So he made up his mind to try to touch base with Bill, Randy's dad. A short time later, they met for lunch. A segment of their conversation follows:

Bill: I'm sorry, Pastor, I haven't been coming to church.

Perry: Oh, no. That's not why I called you.

Bill: What do you mean?

Perry: Well, I hope you don't mind if I ask, but it's about Randy. I hear things . . .

Bill: Of course you can ask me about Randy! But I tell you, Pastor, sometimes I think he's got us all on the run.

Perry: How do you mean? I remember coming to the hospital where we thought things were looking up.

Bill: Not exactly. He's been in the psych ward again, and
             even in jail. He started a fight at a halfway house once,
             and even totally disappeared for weeks on end. Coun-
             selors can't seem to reach him at all . . . sometimes I
             just don't know. Were Jill and I that bad as parents?
             What more can we do? Have we failed?

Perry: Bill, I had no idea. I can sure see you have reason to be
             frustrated. But I wonder if there isn't a difference be-
             tween *failure* and *defeat*. What you've just told me
             doesn't detract a bit from my estimate of you and Jill
             to have been as good parents as any others I know:
             defeated sometimes, but then coming back. Just like
             we learned in sports, don't you think? To *fail* is to have
             given up. OK, maybe defeated, but you folks are
             hardly failures. Nobody over at church or anywhere
             else I know blames you, either, believe me.

Bill: Thanks, Pastor . . . wish Jill could have been here with
             us.

Perry: Well, why not? Let's plan a time. . . .

Upon serving the Rivers (minus Randy) family communion on
the Sunday after the visit, Pastor Perry remembered a Bible verse
from the previous day's devotions:

> To make an apt answer is a joy to anyone
> and a word in season, how good it is! (Prov. 15:23)

FRUITS OF REPENTANCE

Neither parent nor pastor had denied or explained away Randy's
behavior. Rather, they had discussed its powers and pledged an
unspoken commitment to counter them. Upon observing his new
neighbors at Umphumulo Seminary, our African benefactor had
gone a step further and offered a specific response to our need. With
Randy, however, support giving would be far more difficult and
complicated to determine. Only a new relationship challenging
prejudice, negotiated in risk and built upon patience, would do.

For many the term "negotiation" means labor dispute activity
with anticipated dialogue representing opposing viewpoints. It will

also suggest the exciting prospect of taking a fast hairpin turn on the road. A broader, humanistic spin to the word entails the notion of personal change and adaptability.[4] This interpretation best clarifies Pastor Perry's decision to question his own long-held opinions and bear witness to those suffering from mental illness and its consequences in the First Church family.

By the term "mental," I refer to diseases that affect the brain, emotions, and someone's ability to accommodate the usual personal and employment tasks. For Chaplain Vanderzee, negotiation necessitates a process by which "patient, family and physician become collaborators in the struggle of learning how to live with chronic illness."[5] It will produce a dynamic give-and-take exchange wherein the physician pays more attention to the patient's and family's experience of the illness; then in turn they pay more attention to the doctor's point of view. Consider several leads for negotiating pastoral care for such families.

On a broader scale, sympathy for the heartaches confronting families with members having disabilities comes first. American ideology today still extols healthy family units turning out mental health achievers in the area of self-fulfillment and sufficiency. Children are expected to meet specified milestones of progress (especially in education) to accomplish the independence and autonomy expected in our culture.[6] Pastors willing to discuss these expectations with a critical eye can help families exhibiting anxieties about falling behind. When Pastor Perry looked beyond new member recruitment and the success stories he had heard so often he decided to promote contacts with marginal church members such as the Rivers and other "disabled" families. They might have told him "no thanks" in a desire for privacy. Moreover, pastors should recognize that families out of touch with church ministry are by no means always pitiable or helpless. They may already have a support network in place made up of professionals, friends, and relatives, or similarly stressed families in their local NAMI (National Alliance for the Mentally Ill) chapter. This did not happen to be the case with the Rivers. Refusing to ignore rebuffs or defeats, pastors offering sympathy become the foundation for negotiating care.

Health ideology implicates a second discussion area in moving toward caring. Current attitudes revere science and its power to cure disease; most of us assume an eventual laboratory antidote for every sickness in any circumstance. Crisis calls fit into this power theme. As a consequence, chronic sufferers—embarrassments to the vision—are left on the margins. I summon pastors also to pursue faithfully the "chronic" call and to grow more sensitive in thinking about *care* in the absence of *cure*. Shun the *indifference* that hides behind the "busyness" excuse.

Abundant life (see John 10:10) pulses even in our illnesses. In their aftermath pastors with a heart may learn to stimulate conversation about earlier times and life story accounts; they will also try to facilitate better collaboration with physicians and other professionals who may even themselves long for such communication.

A third pastoral care potential I envision incorporates theology. The family may become jaded by futile medical and psychosocial language overload. Bible texts or references to resources of prayer and Christian fellowship will have been carefully avoided in it. Yet, what is distinctive and unique about the Gospel applies to all defeats. Thus, one's spiritual language, reflection, and prayer must more than ever undergird pastoral initiative and negotiations. (See next chapter.) Having prayerfully thought more about one's distinctive spiritual authority and resources should promote the courage to act upon them.

Finally, the attitudes pastors encounter concerning people with disabilities in general are important to initiating dialogue. Common words we use here require careful interpretation. *Impairment* (resulting in loss) forms the basic identity of this minority group. *Disability*, in turn, refers to losses of function as a consequence and most often affects employment opportunities. A handicap is the imposed social perception of the "physically challenged." Consider the results: broadly classified people bearing skeletal anomalies (paralyzed limbs or using wheelchairs) are pitied as *victims*. Those with hearing and vision difficulties (sensory impairments) are considered "less than" and assigned degrees of *helplessness*. Finally, emotionally disturbed individuals are feared as *threats*. This estimate can become the heaviest cross of all.

Pastoral care entails sifting reality from fantasy in each of these arenas.[7] For example, someone is not *confined* to a wheelchair; he or she simply *uses* one. Another person is "on medication" but the treatment hardly disqualifies him or her from attending college classes or poses any danger to others. By mutual respect for language boundaries pastors, patients, medics, and family caregivers can better negotiate reality in their changed and changing worlds.

EMPATHY

Today more than ever I take notice of foreign guests on the campus where I teach. There have been visiting professors from Africa, India, and the People's Republic of China. My own exposure to overseas teaching adds to this new sensitivity; I recall moments when, far from home and loved ones, anxieties and waves of loneliness arose. How meaningful, then, were the gifts from the Umphumulo caretaker who sympathized. Hence in recent years Alice and I have taken note of foreigners and invited them for tourist outings and meals in our home. Efforts to care were not burdensome; to the contrary, we have delighted in the fellowship.

When sympathy grows and moves beyond recognizing predicaments of others to the edges of their experience itself, another term helps us understand negotiation tie-ins. A "feeling into"—empathy—accepts the concerns of others. Moreover, whereas sympathy may mean "I want to help you," empathy arouses the feeling "I *am* you."[8] Persons and sometimes objects can stir our feelings and make us pause: a prairie sunset or the sign-holder at the freeway confronting traffic with "Will work for food" suggest current examples. Or look back upon the empathy of John Donne's meditation:

> No man is an island, entire of itself; every man is a piece of the continent, a part of the main. . . . Any man's death diminishes me, because I am involved in mankind; and therefore never send to know for whom the bell tolls; it tolls for thee.[9]

And only men and women—not machines, pills, or CT scans—can provide care of this nature for hospital patients. Physicians will acknowledge neglect of empathy in current medical practice. Having been reared on educational competition, they learn that victories come through hard work and professionalism. And applause comes through treatment employing objective scientific facts leading to cure. But what if things do not seem to work out that way? Empathy for the defeated, the humble, and the dying hardly fits in this atmosphere. Not everyone wins the race. One man, down with pneumonia, shrank from his jolly, confident physicians. They were too healthy for him.[10]

Pastors in affluent congregations may also admit to the lure of success: new members, budget growth, and compliments from "achieving" parishioners. The less affluent, the abused, and the forgotten ones can come later. Beyond the soup kitchens the challenge for negotiating attention for "least" members like Randy Rivers (see Matt. 25:31-46) remains. But how? Is empathy a gift or a skill? No simple answers suffice when the Randys of the world resist and reject "traditional religion."

Revising cherished "success" attitudes could establish a starting place.[11] Negotiate a stance between too much emotional involvement on the one hand and detachment and distancing on the other. Let biblical narrative compete with cultural fads for attention. Study accounts of persons in the Bible led by the Spirit and try to respect intuition as well as cold facts and reason. It could enhance community, church, and professional contacts to begin a process of better support for those needing it most. Try always to keep in mind what one observer notes:

> When one has surgery or develops a physical illness, people come to visit, to express sympathy, to raise spirits, and to encourage recovery. Such support, we know, has therapeutic value, as does the opportunity to share troubling experiences with others. When an individual has a mental disorder and fears the effects of disclosure, however, he or she does not have the same access to, or expectation of, empathic support.[12]

Yet negotiating care goes both ways, too. In fact, research reports that of those citizens who seek relief from emotional problems, nearly half turn to clergy first.[13] And many unsung benefits ensue.

Young Mark Talbot had already tasted life behind locked hospital doors for mental disorder treatment. And he had no intention of returning even amidst the familiar signs of relapse in his household. Finally, his parents, Joe and Ginny, called their minister. To their enormous relief, he talked Mark into changing his mind about returning to the psych ward voluntarily.[14]

But upon release and potential relapse, what then? After acute-stage contacts like these, "chronic" ministry with family sufferers could continue by challenging public stigma and stereotypes, beginning in the congregation. Informed communicating in preaching and teaching can mediate a vital pastoral presence.

PART II:
MEDIATOR

Persons came to him [Jesus] in their depleted condition, and they left with every reason in the world to be hopeful for the foreseeable—and unforeseeable—future.

Donald Capps
Agents of Hope

We are ambassadors for Christ, since God is making his appeal through us.

2 Cor. 5:20

Chapter 5

Telling the Truth

People with schizophrenia are frequently labeled as "schizo-phrenics," persons with psychosis are "psychotics," and so forth. Use of such terms in this way subtly dehumanizes the afflicted person, implying that the disorders define *the individual rather than describe a fluctuating or temporary psychiatric condition.*

Otto F. Wahl
Media Madness: Public Images of Mental Illness

Following contact and personal familiarity with the private hells brought on by severe and chronic mental illness, the pastor may begin to share the sadness as an empathetic guest in the family circle.

Confronting isolation and providing community come next. Working as a team of sorts, this means caregivers and family members starting efforts to "go public" for everyone concerned. When and how this occurs will vary with each family situation. Important to add here is Herbert Anderson's insight that, for the most part, learning how to work with families is more a matter of perspective than a matter of intervention.[1] Yet if, for example, gossip pins the cause of mental illness exclusively upon poor parenting or drug abuse, the "team" will spring into action and challenge the stereotype on the spot.

Prejudice, stigma, and gossip notwithstanding, however, every pastor can take the first step toward finding this sought-after community by telling the truth at a site perhaps least expected: the pulpit.

THE STING OF FLIPPANCY

"SCHIZ-O-PHRE-NIA, the split mind . . . " intones the radio preacher, "shrinks can make a fortune by giving mind-numbing drugs as the answer." The solution, then? "Come to Jesus. All you need is Jesus!" Ridicule and ignorance aside, our subject requires validity and simple fairness in "speaking the truth in love . . . " (Eph. 4:15). It can also provoke a review of preaching habits and sermon preparation. Jesus invested much effort in teaching. Yet he also preached the Gospel:

> Now after John was arrested, Jesus came to Galilee, proclaiming the good news of God, and saying, "The time is fulfilled and the kingdom of God has come near; repent and believe in the good news." (Mark 1:14-15)

Declaring God's message follows proclamation in the Old Testament. Messengers announcing victory over Israel's enemies move King David to tell the "glad news of deliverance in the great congregation" (Psalm 40:9). During the Babylonian Captivity the promise of a *new* exodus frames the prophet's exaltation:

> How beautiful upon the mountains are the feet of the messenger who announces peace, who brings good news, who announces salvation, who says to Zion, "Your God reigns." (Isa. 52:7)

People in the pews today also long for breakthroughs of surprise and hope about the God who reigns. An inspired Christian sermon can make vivid God's gospel in Christ as revealed in the Bible. Through quite human messengers such as ourselves, God's Holy Spirit may call forth faith in God's continuing work in our lives. Families with burdens of chronic illness—stroke, Alzheimer's, mental—will be alert for promises of victory over chaos and evil in hope for God's ultimate rule. From this vantage, preachers and listeners can face life and death with renewed courage, more confident of our God-given dignity. As a consequence, we are moved to distinguish better between the center and the periphery, between the ultimate and the trivial. Preaching takes as ultimately serious the good news as known in Jesus Christ for our salvation and spiritual growth. It becomes *an event* for thirsting listeners.[2] Gratitude, hope, and resolve are born amidst words such as forgiveness, hope, trust, and grace.

How sad, then, to hear incoherent sermons drowning a biblical text in trite personal opinions and "psychobabble." Psychological jargon drenches our culture. The terms ego, self-esteem, stress, and lifestyle are so commonplace few ever try to define them or learn about their more specific use in office or classroom. In a radio sermon I recently heard, the preacher spoke about his pet dog being slightly "paranoid schizophrenic." Another minister announced his acquaintance with a "schizzie." And psychiatrists will "merely fill you full of pills to drown your sorrows." A recent sermon cited the uselessness of a "gut full of Prozac."[3] Thoughtless scoffing at the medical profession degrades the pulpit.

Privately I have heard what I consider clergy overuse of slang such as "nuts," "crazy," and "psycho." There was even a joke about "deviled ham" in reference to the story discussed earlier about the unclean spirits' banishment to the swine and their subsequent plunge into the sea (Mark 5:11-12 and Luke 8:27-33). Careless and reckless labels are sometimes intended to disparage political opponents. Calling Saddam Hussein a "madman" in a newspaper editorial is not meant as serious analysis; rather, the mental illness label belittles or maligns the leader in a way that subscribers are accustomed to. Yet exaggeration is not the only problem in this case; the real fault lies in the accompanying discredit it conveys to those actually struggling with mental illness, both sufferers and family members alike. Try to imagine other serious or life-threatening illnesses as publicly identified in such fashion. Consider Parkinson's, multiple sclerosis, or cancer. In poor taste, everyone agrees, and totally unacceptable. Slang terms such as "loony," "wacko," and "sicko" are residuals of past unflattering conceptions. Media analyst Otto Wahl cites "lunatic" as a leftover of a time when:

People with mental illnesses were seen as little more than insensate beasts, when they were chained and treated as objects of amusement for nobles who paid to view them as in a human zoo.[4]

Having had first-hand observations of situations involving both paranoia and schizophrenia (as defined by medics), it makes me wince to hear such trivializing of human suffering. What if families of people facing heart disease in loved ones were treated this way? (Any jokes about cancer or bypass operations out there?) Such carelessness betrays both clergy ignorance and arrogance. And since congregation members also look up to their ministers for biblical insight and consider their address as worthy of trust, the damage deepens. So unthinking clergy can thus become engaged in establishing harmful falsehoods, even though unintended. To add to the sad package, superficial opinions will plant themselves only too readily. Remember that words such as "foolish," "silly," "stupid," or "bizarre" can still identify unacceptable fashion or behavior. No one need surrender honesty.

Nor need we forsake humor. To a tourist visitor, formal Sunday church attendance in Scandinavia often appears sparse. Thus I chuckled recently at this "question and answer":

- How do you define "paranoia"?
- You're sitting in the front row during a Danish Lutheran Church service and you think there is someone behind you!

Can we "lighten up" in coping without ridiculing? Yes, and I affirm its value especially for the caregiver in the long run.

In our popular culture, the metaphor of illness used to describe all sorts of anxieties, discomforts, or deviant behaviors as needing psychiatric attention has become commonplace. Persons and families are "addicted" or "dysfunctional." But such talk diverts attention from the severe problems facing the chronically mentally ill and their families as described earlier. Pastors can at least resist this damaging tendency by refusing to add to it with superficial references in public discourse: "Things can get so bad," it slips out, "that sometimes you wonder if you'll be able to maintain your sanity." Mental illness may involve a brain disease. Will the health of a person diagnosed with cancer be maintained simply by an act of will, important as this is? It makes me want to leave church by the back door.

FAITHFULLY SILENT

Our world is so full of noise—traffic, jet blasts, blaring televisions—that it seems at times modern culture wants to avoid even an appearance of silence. Yet with biblical backgrounds we can remember incidents of stillness. David's resistance to his "outside" world turns the poet inward: "For God alone my soul waits in silence . . ." (Psalm 62:1). The author of Ecclesiastes declares "a time to keep silence" (Eccles. 3:7). Jesus kept silence before his accusers (Mark 14:61). Such reminders suggest how silence can lead to a special kind of inner stillness today as well. An achievement of an inner strength may create a spiritual resource to keep one's "ego needs" more in check or possibly to endure hidden pain. Silence within may prove inadequate or inappropriate. During times of acute or long-term suffering so many of us cannot seem to "find words." After a SIDS (sudden infant death syndrome) incident, an impending divorce situation, or a job downsizing, a "what can I say?" pause so often surrounds us as a symbol of surrender. But as one observer notes, eventually *context* will make a difference: we must ask, within what kind of relationship is silence maintained? Which person maintains it? Is there a conscious purpose for it, like feelings of guilt or shame?[5]

While respecting periods of "living in silence" with others, I advocate promoting an intentional, nontrivializing posture of reaching out instead. Such a stance eventually can find community even in the face of silent answers to the perpetual question "Why?" and open up to others under the broader agenda of human suffering. Consider the following example:

In his book, *Living with Chronic Illness*, Stephen A. Schmidt—himself encountering long-term disability—discusses the question, old as the biblical Job's, "Why did this happen to me?" He concludes:

> No, God doesn't relieve the illness. No, I am not about to receive a miracle. . . . Yes, I believe God loves me—now, in this mess. . . . No, I do not understand why these things happen to me. Yes, I have hope. Yes, I have faith. So we say yes, no, yes. Mystery. Surely there are clues. . . . But ultimately I am left silent, faithfully silent.[6]

Sometimes pastoral caregivers can also succumb to a "What can I add?" attitude. Furthermore, if they do attempt language of support, as novice learners they can find themselves caught between *disease* talk (as defined medically) and *patienthood* (as defined socially) language contexts. Yet they are considered professionals nonetheless, expected to deal with a complex range of life situations involving "waiting room" clientele now certified by society as patients. Moreover, well-intended helpers will meet their "children of God" parishioners who are often angry, puzzled, and disenchanted by being forced to make plans involving unpleasant choices. Sometimes silence seems best. P.W. Pryser's contention, however, upholds a positive distinctiveness of the pastor's role at this point:

> In a word, pastors represent a profession that does something to suffering by placing it in a unique perspective that addresses its omnipresence, its possible meanings, its roles in life, its impact on people's integrity, its ultimate origins, and its ultimate implications.[7]

To follow through on Pryser's confidence in care potentials of pastors, let me review the family situation as framed in previous chapters:

Discovering the Family Burden

Contexts

1. Spouse, siblings
2. Parent-child
3. "Chronic" (long-term, serious, challenging), acute and recovery stages

Burden Stimulants

1. Behavioral aspects of the illness
   a. Annoying or threatening behavior
   b. Alienating family members
   c. Provoking empathetic pain in other family members
2. Quandaries
   a. Behavior: out of control or not?
   b. Independence: an impossible dream?
   c. Best treatment plans, degree of care?

Burden: Overviews, Past, and Present

1. Family as agents of causality, of rehabilitation
2. Long-term strains
   a. Tolerance or spiritual growth?
   b. Bereavement, grief, and mourning

Basic Trends

1. Confused images of health (families and mental health professionals)
2. Growing acceptance of biological aspects of the illness, continuing education

BREAKING THE SILENCE

The "how to" of deciding to care about mental illness affairs flows from this posture; prayerful study with dependence upon the Spirit's lead can enable healing responses to the unique challenges of a given contact.

Theological distinctiveness and confidence will emerge, first of all, with time in the study to discover more about psychiatry and suffering. Two resources are indispensable:

1. E. Fuller Torrey, *Surviving Schizophrenia: A Manual for Families, Consumers and Providers*, Third edition (New York: Harper Perennial, 1995). Topics include diagnosis of mental illness, treatment, rehabilitation, major problems, and advocacy. First-rate expertise in layperson language qualifies this as a "Bible" for the serious researcher.
2. Rodney J. Hunter, H. Newton Malony, Liston O. Mills, John Patton, eds. *Dictionary of Pastoral Care and Counseling* (Nashville: Abingdon Press, 1990). Links with theological topics are found in articles such as "Salvation, Healing and Health" plus "Faith Healing" and "Religion and Health." If Torrey is the Bible, the *Dictionary* becomes St. Augustine, plus a bit of Martin Luther and the Talmud.

Suppose you attend a service club or conference meeting where a speaker employs language such as, "Have you ever felt a bit paranoid about crime and those weirdos out on the street?" or "What kind of schizophrenic society do we have, anyway?" Having done a bit of homework in the above resources, you could politely ask for further definition of terms such as paranoid. My guess is that you would encounter serious misunderstandings and at the same time open avenues for truth and advocacy.

A second context for breaking the silence will entail biblical studies and eventual sermon preparation. It might also mean revising trite talk about "demons" and current culture. With your personal favorite study resources of theological word book, atlas, and commentary at hand, let's return (see Chapter 1) to the country of the Gerasenes, this time with Mark's account:

Demons, Then and Now (Mark 5:1-20)

Study Guide Questions

1. Note verses 1-5. Is the man a "raving maniac?" Does "lunatic fringe" define his behavior and habitat? Compare deinstitutionalization then and now.
2. Verses 6-7. The possessed man represents opposition to God's voice (the "adversary" of I Peter 5:8?). See also Genesis 3 and concordance for references to "devil," "Satan," and "evil one."
3. Verses 8-13. Consult commentaries and J. Moltmann, *The Way of Jesus Christ*, 108-112, to interpret the exorcism. Which of the following terms best helps clarify these verses: miracle, healing, or power? Why?
4. Verses 14-15. What characterizes "right mind" here? In our society? Is psychotherapy today's exorcism?
5. Why the *fear* of Jesus (vs. 15) and the request to leave their neighborhood (vs. 17)? Compare with NIMBY ("not in my back yard") anxieties about group residence plans to house deinstitutionalized mental patients. Relate "mercy" to Leviticus 19:18 and to our congregation.
6. Design a sermon outline from the man's reformed voice (vs. 20).

7. Take another look at the Pryser quotation on p. 62. Is *hope* the key to understanding it better? See Donald Capps, *Agents of Hope: A Pastoral Psychology.* For additional counsel note "Family Concerns and the Silence of the Pulpit" in Elizabeth Achtemeier's *Preaching about Family Relationships*, 9-16.
8. Is it ignorance or mockery? "A neurotic builds castles in the sky. A psychotic lives in them. A psychiatrist collects the rent!"[8]
9. How would you respond to a sermon stating that "medication does no good; the devil and demons need to be thrown out."[9]
10. Discuss: Is good health, including sanity, the purpose of life? (Relate your thoughts to discipleship.) Health idolatry: real or imagined? See Ephesians 6:10-17.

TESTING THE AMBIGUITIES

Luke's Social World, Then and Now (Luke 8:26-29)

Compare and contrast the emphasis:[10]

Gerasene Country	Today's America
• Being and becoming	• Doing
• Relationships	• The autonomous self, individual preference
• Nature uncontrollable	• Manipulation or mastery of nature
• Human nature as both good and bad	• Human nature as neutral or correctable

Discovering Ministry

In 1990, I conducted a survey study and received 142 responses from family members acquainted with our subject.[11] On the familiar scale of 1 to 10 (with 10 as the highest value), the directions asked, "As a family member having experienced the effects of mental illness you can help by circling the appropriate number for each of the options listed." The results were as follows:

Clergy, Congregation, and Mental Illness

		Score
1.	Counsel on family stability and marital tensions	8.2
2.	Preaching that includes words such as "paranoid" and "schizophrenia"	6.1
3.	Help in dealing with guilt, shame, and embarrassment	8.7
4.	Promoting adult religious education about chronic mental illness	9.1
5.	Noncondemning acceptance of family anger and frustration	9.3
6.	Information about such treatment options as community mental health centers	9.3
7.	Encouragement to "tell our stories"	8.5
8.	Clergy calling at the hospital during acute stages	7.7
9.	Clergy should ignore chronic and family aspects	2.7
10.	Congregations should encourage persons with mental illness to attend public worship	8.3

Each of us can contribute special insights by responding to these questions and ambiguities. As a result, at least ridicule and carelessness about mental illness should fade from sermons; we may even share the results of our discoveries through spiritual growth and find ourselves as even more authentic ambassadors for Christ in the process (2 Cor. 5:20). One thing is certain from the survey: clergy are needed and wanted.

Formal Christian education presents a different and more wide-open opportunity for changing the community Otto Wahl cites in this chapter's epigraph. I turn, then, from the pulpit to the lectern or to those places having less formal circles of seekers and learners.

Chapter 6

Teaching the Congregation

A church can intentionally educate its members about mental illness. It can teach what mental illness is; what the characteristics are; how it can be treated; and how to eliminate myths about mental illness.

S. Duane Bruce
Caring Congregations

She decided to accept the challenge. Barbara, pastor of a small but growing suburban church, would organize the topic of mental illness for the agenda of next fall's adult education forum.

Months earlier, she had received a crisis phone call from a parent whose son dropped out of college in mid-term to obtain psychiatric care. The young minister had known Tim slightly from youth activities but this turn of events was totally unexpected. A visit to the psychiatric ward shocked and saddened her. Later on, after hearing about Tim's suicide attempt, Barbara felt more helpless than ever when it came to ministering to the young man's family.

During one of her visits to St. Mary's she spoke of her bewilderment to the hospital chaplain, Dick. He passed along a brochure advertising a free workshop series soon to be offered by the local community mental health center titled, "Mental Health Mondays." One of the sessions, "When a Loved One Has a Mental Illness," promised to focus on how mental illness affects the family. Others, such as "It's Monday . . . Are You Depressed?" aroused her curiosity.

The pastor made room on her tight schedule. The first workshop evening proved quite stimulating but seemed to raise more questions than answers. The sequel on depression, "It's Wednesday . . .

Are You Still Depressed?" gave the earnest caregiver pause for assessing her own (never mentioned to anyone else) nagging bouts with occasional letdowns occurring mostly after festival seasons during the church year. The instructor responded to Barbara's "Thank you for the session" with a question: "Well, are churches doing anything along these lines? There's so much to do out there."

Let's put ourselves in this pastor's place and go about "doing something" in the face of this summons for better religious education.

BACK TO THE BASICS

These days teachers in the public schools offer a variety of services ranging from monitoring and coaching to reporting signs of child abuse. Important as these activities may be, many parents and other concerned citizens would prefer more focus upon "readin', writin' and 'rithmetic"—the *basics*.

Church members could define a similar lack of focus in parish educational efforts as well. Assuming their claim is generally true, in this chapter, I seek to remind readers of basics meaningful to any Christian leader and especially to the educational ministry of committed pastors such as Barbara. The parish-based setting for such activity is also important. Besides, admitting how introducing somewhat artificial topics can blur our "basics" focus in some instances, I intend nevertheless to suggest the subject of mental illness for congregational learning agendas. It may surprise some that the matter at hand is even in the Bible. But I claim its mysteries can educate all of us into renewed experiences of faith, hope, and love.

Teachers

Parents are primary teachers in the Old Testament. It warns,

> Hear, my child, your father's instruction, and do not reject your mother's teaching; for they are a fair garland for your head, and pendants for your neck. (Prov. 1:8-9)

The verb "to teach" here means not so much an intellectual activity of dispensing information; rather, it signals an invitation to

God and the divine will expressed in the commandments. Both parent and child become involved in hearing, reciting, discussion, and devotional obedience to them (Deut. 6:4-9; 11:18-20). Following Moses, the rabbi teaches disciples the will of God based upon tradition and the sacred writings.

Education in the ancient Greek world—so influential still—departed somewhat from such an emphasis upon the total personality. Here teachers stressed the mind in the exercise of reason, the body in the case of sport, and skills in the case of art techniques.[1] In the New Testament gospels "rabbi" or "teacher" is the title most commonly given to Jesus and reference to his teaching activity appears some fifty times in the texts. Eventually the disciples become active collaborators in mission (Mark 1:17; 3:14-15).[2]

Later, the terms "pastor" and "teacher" are joined together in Ephesians (4:11). Pastoral care embodies both the Jewish and Greek heritage of thought and action. The outcome balances skill and art in an ever-open process. A prominent Christian educator writes:

> If the church is to be worthy of its divine origin, it does not stand still, but must always advance into new areas. Each pastor is potentially a teacher.[3]

Pastoral caregivers not only will promote a "holistic" empathy for families suffering as a consequence of mental illness, they will also insist that members of the flock *think* about the social status of their incapacitated loved ones. As a result they will become more effective educators (Latin: "to lead forth") themselves. And for this reason especially, teaching pastors will join their inquirers as "leading learners" and agents of vision.[4]

Learners

Children and adolescents are sometimes very much a part of the family burdens described in previous chapters. Yet the learners, whom visionary clergy will lead in bringing to light more about them, are mostly adults; thus the needs—educationally speaking—of middle-aged and older parishioners become paramount.

As a college teacher I have noticed in recent years a shift upward in the student age level from an accustomed norm of eighteen- to twenty-two-year-olds. These days a class can include adults such as a retired Air Force officer, a single parent who sometimes brings her child along, and someone who, having lost employment, seeks to upgrade credentials. More than ever, middle-aged and older adults offer lively contributions to class discussions.

Implying a teaching ministry, Jesus commands Peter to "feed my lambs" and "tend my sheep" (John 21:15-16). Learners today as sheep and lambs? The picture hardly fits. Visitors to Australia and New Zealand witness flocks of sheep turned into cowering and obedient "mobs" by innocuous little dogs. It doesn't connect with my classes at all. Yet in the context of the Master Teacher's "I am the good shepherd. The good shepherd lays down his life for the sheep" (John 10:11), we can appreciate that the metaphor's point is human vulnerability and our total dependence upon God's power to save and renew.

How, then, should we characterize today's adult learner? First on my list concerns time. As the passage of years seems to accelerate with the death of parents, relatives, and friends, so does the appreciation for the finality of time. A child or young adult measures years as "time since birth" whereas an adult past forty measures years as "time until death."[5] Adults in Christian education classes have little interest in storing information for possible use at a later date. This insight relates to a second earmark: these learners are more problem-centered than subject-centered. I visited recently with a young adult couple enthused about the previous week's Community Sunday forum at their church. A guest speaker had introduced the topic, "Violence in Society—What Can We Do About It?" and had given them something to think about. Caring for elderly parents, to mention another example, becomes more immediate than issues of peace and nuclear war. The first two illustrations open up a better path for decision making and action than the other, more unmanageable subject. Because in the day when communication brings issues of our society and the world into one's living room, a third trait of adult learners is the potential of such lay persons to join visionary "leading learner" clergy in creative response to change and emerging issues in the Church's mission.

THE LIBEL OF OUR LABELS

In previous chapters I have profiled current medical and social contexts of mental illness and traced their impact upon families. Can parish-based clergy make a difference? Yes! Pastoral care framed within a congregational teaching ministry is one way.

As a young pastor, I served a four-congregation parish. It not only required much time on the road but also, I soon discovered, myriad administrative duties: getting out the bulletin, checking into furnace repair, and so on. Looking back, the only adults I taught were in new member classes; challenging other adult learners in thinking over a Christian response to current issues slipped completely off my priority list. I suspect pastors today face similar situations, even more so in an urbanizing society featuring rising crime statistics, domestic violence, youth on drugs, spiraling divorce rates, and other disturbing trends.

For the renewing of our minds as Christians "we have gifted persons . . . " writes the Apostle—ministers, pep talk artists, philanthropists, caregivers—as well as "the teacher in teaching . . . " (Rom. 12:2, 7-8).

Self-Study

After determining to imitate the Mental Health Mondays workshops of her local mental health center at church, Pastor Barbara wondered how to begin. I advocate adding a "Christ and mental illness" workshop to the pastoral care self-study agenda.

A community mental health center visit with time spent amidst client activities there would illuminate treatment from a usually hidden local ally. In addition, I trust the previous chapters will help equip parish-based nonspecialist clergy with basic understandings. Continuing education courses, audio-visual materials, and a host of other reading titles could maintain the learning.

Questions more than answers stimulate self-study initiatives. Try to imagine conversations and materials. Then, later on, discuss your opinions with others.

Consider:

1. Are some prophetic actions "psychotic"? (Ezek. 3:24-25; 4:4 ff; 24:15 ff) And Jesus? (Mark 3:11; 19b-21 and John 7:20; 10:20) Why or why not?
2. Recall Jonestown (1978), Waco, Texas, David Koresh and, more recently, the "Heaven's Gate" suicides. Does "apocalyptic religion" contribute to mental disorder?
3. Distinguish between neurosis and eccentricity. Apply to American "speaking in tongues" and snake-handling activities.
4. Would you like to visit a "psych" ward? Why or why not?
5. Does the religious educator addressing mental illness model mental *health* for others at the same time?
6. What is the difference between hallucination-delusion terminology and biblical dreams and visions?
7. Do we erase stigma or merely manage it? (Think of terms such as schizzie, crazy, nuts, weirdo, wacko, loony, and psycho.)
8. In our industrial society, we seem to have more mental illness than in preindustrial societies. Why?
9. A recovering patient comments, "Jesus expelled demons. Why doesn't he expel mine?" How would you reply?
10. A recent study reveals that whereas four percent of persons with serious mental illness have violent tendencies, 77 percent of portrayals in the media refer to the tendency. Is media bashing justified?

Conversational feedback to these questions will succeed better when three rules are agreed upon:

1. In some instances let questions remain questions.
2. Agree to disagree at times but look up additional information resources.
3. From changed attitudes, work together for an active response of specific services.

Research in religious education shows that the primary quality needed for overall pastoral effectiveness corresponds to rule #3. Congregations appreciate especially those pastors who assist laity to take up their own ministries.[6] Examples of current models are found in the next chapter.

Apprentices

Parishioners value pastoral ties with their congregation's leader in spite of new gods of technology and leisure created by twentieth-century culture. Many adult learners anticipate a "time before death" pilgrimage more than ever and want to understand best how to serve beyond assisting at the altar and taking up the collection. Fashioning such Christians now requires instruction, education, and what Stanley Hauerwas and John Westerhoff describe as "formation":

> Instruction informs us in terms of knowledge and skills believed by the community to be important for communal life. Education reforms us by aiding us to discover dissonance between how we are living and how we are called to live. And formation both conforms (nurtures) and transforms (converts) us through a process best understood as apprenticeship.[7]

Forming a healing response to persons with mental illness and their family members coping with various burdens demands various levels of apprenticeship from anyone. So I continue with a discussion starter outline designed for a beginner's adult class series. Let me introduce the background for the effort.

Auditory hallucination—hearing voices—is a primary diagnostic characteristic of schizophrenia. They may be swishing or thumping sounds, a single voice repeating incoherent words (Why not? . . . Be it . . . Why, if . . . Why? . . . Because I . . .) without context, or even the voices of a choir. In the vast majority of cases they are unpleasant, reviling victims for past misdeeds either real or imagined.[8] It's enough to "drive a person crazy," isn't it? Let's accept this instruction from the well-known psychiatrist, E. Fuller Torrey, and move on to complement our learning through Bible study.

First, I suggest an informational approach (vs. a series announcement) for recruiting companion apprentice learners. Newspapers commonly report violent crimes. After citing gruesome details of violence, a journalist often describes the criminal suspect as one with "a history of mental problems." (Why not link the crime to intolerable, evil, wicked, malicious, atrocious, or dangerous drug-induced behavior instead?) The pastor could arouse interest by attending coffee hour fellowship with such a clipping and invite interested folks to join him or her in the corner to talk about it. Questions arise from such articles themselves: What would Jesus say to the victims and the perpetrators of the crime? (See John 8:1-11.) Is your own neighborhood becoming more violent? What about domestic violence? Are Christians responsible for changing things? and so on. Members of the circle would be invited to bring their own clippings and further musings along for the following Sunday.

Eventually a consensus will form around queries, such as, What does the Bible say about evil? What about demons, and so much violence, especially in the Old Testament? By now the companion researchers should be more receptive for a "leading learner" pastor's teaching ministry.

Next, I offer several additional clusters of study and conversation guidelines centered around the schizophrenic "hearing voices" symptom. I employ the Bible as the basic text, respect the community of learning in a Christian congregation, and utilize Hauerwas and Westerhoff's threefold description of teaching.

HEARING VOICES: YOUR NEIGHBOR'S CHRONIC MENTAL ILLNESS

Acquiring a Voice

The first cluster sets forth information about the illness (select from Chapter 1, "The Challenge," or the second chapter, "Family Impact") and its current appearances in our society. Consult resources listed in the Appendix.

The intention is to enable informed opinions to begin with. A stimulant for discussion (gaining a "voice") with opinions that are open for revision, continued learning, and potential empathy come later.

Listening

1. "Defeated" parishioners
2. Mental health professionals in congregation
3. National Alliance for the Mentally Ill, chaplains
4. Attention, not cure (vs. isolation)

Learning

1. Literature
2. Medical model, community mental health centers

God's Voice

1. In creation (Gen. 1:3, 6, 9, etc. See a Concordance for further citations)
2. For covenant making in human life (Gen. 12, Abraham; Exod. 3, Moses; Exod. 20, Num. 7:89, Deut. 4:6, 15:5)
3. The voice of meaning and order—love to God and neighbors, Luke 10:25-28
4. Issues
   a. Defining neighbors and community
   b. The commandments (Torah) today: losing influence?

Lifting Your Voice

Beyond "Gatekeeper" Counseling

1. Hearing consumer (clients of the mental health system) responses
2. Prayer, Bible study, ritual: superficialities?
3. God's forgiveness, sovereignty, and unconditional love

Teaching

1. Conversation, not explanation
2. "Demon" texts: through, not around disturbing comparisons with mental illness

3. Medication: necessary but not sufficient
4. Stigma confrontation and management

Education

A search to discover differences between our calling to discipleship and our actual efforts and accomplishments. Coping with dissonance by envisioning reform. Our voices and other voices from the Bible.

Other Voices

1. Emotional (illustrations: Esau, Gen. 27:50; anxiety, Jer. 25:8-14; sorrow, Psalm 22)
2. Prayer (Hagar's boy, Gen. 21:17; Prov. 2:3; Psalm 64:1)
3. Prophetic judgment (Jer. 11:1-5)
4. Enthusiasm (the anonymous woman, Luke 11:27)
5. Demonic possession and unclean spirits (Mark 1:21-28 and over seventy other references in the New Testament)

Awaiting the Voice

Formation

1. Nurturing individual and group health in the Church's mission. Avoiding health idolatry. Ministry beyond healing in daily faithfulness to God's unfolding promises. The voice of triumph (Rev. 21:3-4). Healing as conquest of Satan and illness together with promotion of health (Luke 13:10-17).
2. Jesus de-demonizes illness to preserve social relationships (Mark 5:19, "Go home to your friends . . .") and human dignity.
3. Prayerful, eschatological spirituality (John 5:24); brokering patience; ministry *to* becoming ministry *with* (and from? Matt. 25:40, the "least" of these).
4. Personal (temporal) and cosmic (eternal) salvation (John 5:25 and Matt. 28:20). God's power moving toward a new creation (Gen. 1, 2; Rev. 21:1), a "new heaven and earth." A source for rehabilitation and hope.

Questions

1. In terms of congregational ministry link Rev. 21:1 and 1 Cor. 15:57-58. How do we "know"? (vs. 58).
2. Consider such ministry in the perspective of deinstitutionalized, homeless, and marginalized citizens of our neighborhoods.
3. Is "neighbor" defined more by geography or by sharing common interests?

BRIDGE BUILDERS

Marks of the burdens borne by families of persons suffering from symptoms of chronic mental illness may eventually become visible to relatives and close friends. Many will join them in caregiving. In neighborhood congregations worshippers pray, *"Our* Father who art in heaven . . ." and affirm faith's community base. I appeal to this "extended family" for a careful look at the public shadowlands of shame revealed in previous chapters.

From a grassroots level, faithful Christians who choose to care enough will challenge false stereotypes and educate others through new ministries. They can become bridge builders to coordinate private and public spheres of service. Members of the wider family may also help shift intervention from efforts solely devoted to *curing* to actions of *caring* in chronic or long-term visitations of illness.

Religious witness in the public square ordinarily comes to our attention through symbols (buildings and steeples), events (celebrations of Hanukkah and Christmas), and professional ministries (clergy and laypersons). When both shoulder their "leading learner" opportunities, the most effective testimony of its merit arises: informed and faithful parishoners who prove the truth of our Lord's teaching by becoming "salt" and "light" (Matt. 5:13-14).

The next chapter examines strategies and offers illustrations of ministries already underway.

PART III:
ADVOCATE

Until the day break,
and the shadows flee away.

Song of Solomon 2:17 (KJV)

In a sense, then, Christianity, liberal or conservative,
symbolic or liberal, has a basic problem with associating
mental illness with sin, a problem that in practical terms
has been resolved by rendering the afflicted unto Caesar.

Paul J. Fink and Allan Tasman (Eds.)
Stigma and Mental Illness

Chapter 7

Willing to Care

Let's make our congregations places where the persistently mentally ill and their families are truly included. Let's minister to them when they have needs; let's minister with them in deeds of loving kindness; let's search for ways to include ministry by them in what we do.

H. Newton Malony
Paper presented at
The Faith Community and Mental Illness:
Breaking Bread Together conference

Previous chapters have invited readers to become more observant of the illness situation surrounding mental disorder in both individuals and families. We also continue a search for a spiritual framework in this environment. Consequently, now is the time to look beyond individuals, health professionals, and family to another piece of the puzzle, namely, the Christian congregation; this moves us more from description to prescription, from discussing the suffering to the search for practical responses. First we need to remind ourselves about the increasing educational level and great *potential volunteer* make-up within a given congregation of God's people. Discipleship in the train of Christ's own challenge becomes its public mark (John 13:34-35), and discovering contexts for special needs belongs in this effort. Three of them are important here: first, serving more effectively the current situation; second, recognizing contexts for new ministry initiatives; and, finally, learning from and adapting to current models of congregational inclusion of persons with persistent mental illness and their families.

AT THE MANOR

Befriending residents of a group or board and care home presents an immediate context for innovative ministry. These supported living centers have come about from the promise of "community-based care" resulting from the deinstitutionalization of the 1960s. As a typical example, let's name one of them "Mina's Manor." This motel-like structure houses a dozen or so individuals. They receive monthly federal Supplemental Security Income (SSI) checks which—as arranged by the local mental health center—they turn over to the manager who provides a room, three meals a day, and an organized, disciplined day care regimen. This means, for example, that even though one is free to leave at any time, residents report schedules and absences and appear on time for meals. Absences might be due to trips taken for activities sponsored by the local community mental health center (CMHC).

But plenty of free time—especially on weekends—remains on the docket. At Mina's Manor, Sundays are free. During a postbreakfast smoke and second cup of coffee, residents may sit around outside, weather permitting. Should someone arrive with a tray of pastries from the nearby bakery just then, the hour would become special indeed. Upon first checking this out with the manager, delivery volunteers could thereby easily create a neighborhood link between congregation and group home. Eventually, volunteers might linger to swap life stories and perhaps share a hobby. And adult Christian education classes arranged at the Manor might include slides, video interpretations, and Bible studies as well. Residents, shy at first, mostly welcome outsiders and conversation beyond television watching.

Of course, invitations to church belong in these contacts, too. One minister shares his experience of reaching out:

> We have forty board and care homes in our area. Ten of them are in the shadow of our steeple. There are about a hundred people within a mile or two of our steeple living in those homes. Our congregation worked with staff from the South Carolina State Department of Mental Health. They brought a few people from the board and care homes to meet us. They

mingled with us. People who were frightened of people with a mental illness saw they are not a threat to any of us.[1]

It proved to be the beginning of a relationship (for seven years to date) in which group home folks have gradually learned and been encouraged to celebrate events with members of the congregation. "We sing. We dance. We have communion services. Now we bring in people from other congregations."[1] At least for some citizens a concept, namely community-based care for persons with major mental illness, has become reality. And, in this instance, a congregation has led the way.

Besides initiating fellowship with residents in such places as Mina's Manor, a second ministry enterprise could focus upon a congregational adult Christian education interest group. It might emerge as a section of a standing social concerns committee. In any event, I recommend calling the association the Media Watch Committee. To get things started, perhaps at the postservice coffee hour, the pastor could call for attention and simply announce he or she would like to retreat to a corner to discuss a contemporary local crime report concerning an attacker with a "history of mental problems." Or perhaps the topic could be "Demons: Then and Now." After all, Jesus apparently did something of the same when he abruptly called to the crowds, "Listen to me, all of you and understand . . . If any want to become my followers, let them deny themselves and take up their cross" (Mark 7:14; 8:34).

Composed primarily of concerned family members, perhaps a few health professionals, and others with curiosity, Media Watch intentions would feature continuing education plus a resolve to defend the reputation and human dignity of persons "out there" coping with mental illness. The "watch" aspect might invite responses to news items through the Letters to the Editor route. For example, I responded once to the newspapers' use of "schizophrenic" via the following:

To the Editor, *The News Tribune*

Instead of mockery, how about compassion, treatment, and understanding for persons with symptoms of schizophrenia? The patronizing tone of "Acting brings out the schizophrenic in the best of them" (TNT, 1-17) serves to reinforce a cruel stereotyping of persons with mental illness.

Mounting evidence points to a biological basis for mental disorders. This suggests a handicapping condition no more shameful than diabetes or cerebral palsy. And the vast majority of this population is neither violent nor raving in the streets. Furthermore, it is an illness both treatable and curable.

I propose that a more challenging task would be for would-be actors to emulate the "normal" persons around us. It is time to stop treating schizophrenics as the vermin of our society.

SDG Tacoma[2]

On another occasion, a schoolchild reported becoming fearful of the gestures a Fir Lodge Group Home resident had made. A public meeting outcry resulted, which included city government officials. Calls were made for the removal of the home from the neighborhood. It did not happen that way, but my personal advocate media watch committee of one took action again:

To the Editor,
Over the years my contacts with residents of two local Group Homes has shown evidence of law-abiding, generous behavior on the part of these neighbors. Thus I am pleased to note the right of Fir Lodge citizens ("Home for Mentally Ill Will Stay Near School" TNT, October 3, p. B4) has been maintained. Fir Lodge was there *first*.

Smug ignorance, combined with fear-mongering bigotry, will neither resolve misunderstandings nor counter the bombardment of media portrayals stigmatizing mental illness.

At the beginning of Mental Illness Awareness Week (October 6-12), I invite concerned readers to contact one's local community mental health center and the Mental Health Chaplaincy Office of Associated Ministries for information to provide a basis for initiating genuine dialogue.

Sincerely,
SDG[3]

Declaring open season on people suffering from brain disorders also happens through the carelessness of Christians who should know better. For instance, when recently browsing through one of the religious book catalogs so frequently crossing my desk I noted a text devoted to clergy/congregation conflicts. A detail in the promotional blurb triggered another letter to the editor:

> Greetings:
> Thank you for sending me a copy of the new Spring/Summer 1997 catalog. It is attractive and appears to be a valuable resource for my list of yearly department book orders here.
> But on page 28 I was dismayed to see,
>> "Some churches have 'clergy killer' congregations, energized by evil and mentally ill personalities in their midst."
> What?! Persons trying to cope with mental illness are no more evil than the rest of us. And, furthermore, comes the association with "killers." Every day these citizens are slandered in the media as dangerous and violent. Why, I ask, wasn't simply "evil personalities" enough for the blurb? It's bad enough to attempt to manage stigma in the public arena without having it appear among folks who should know better.
> I recognize there are no evil intentions on anybody's part. But if in any way you can counter such a damaging reference many like myself who are involved with ministry and mental disorders will thank you.
>
> Sincerely,
> SDG[4]

In addition to the printed media, the visual also deserves attention. Committee partners could invite their church neighbors to view current (1997) award-winning films such as *Shine* with a critical eye: Was the breakdown and its aftermath plausible? Was the father's role in the onset fairly portrayed?[5] In addition, "classics" such as *Psycho* and *One Flew Over the Cuckoo's Nest* are available.

VOLUNTEER FRIENDSHIP

Providing a church drop-in center for Mina's Manor residents would reach beyond opportunities for church socials and continuing education efforts as described earlier. But the possibility would also mean considerably greater investments of planning time and resources. Continue prayerful reflections about these "shut-outs."

The Compeer Program is another possibility that would perhaps prove more practical and effective in the long run. "Compeer" blends the words companion, equal, and peer. It was born in Rochester, New York, some twenty years ago as an "adopt-a-patient" program with a local mental health facility. From Rochester and serving twelve individuals, Compeer has grown to a world-wide network, the International Affiliation of Compeer Programs (IACP), with affiliates in 119 cities, 28 states, Australia, and Canada. As of 1996, 4,000 consumers of mental health care are being served.

Based on the concept that volunteer friendship and support can offset the isolation and loneliness experienced with mental illness, Compeer acts as a go-between for/with the volunteer, the therapist, and the Compeer friend. It provides respite to coping families as well. Thousands of its promoted friendships build trust, help reaffirm human dignity, and develop self-sufficiency. These are vital components for reentry of deinstitutionalized patients into the mainstream of community life. Volunteers, having been matched with a possible new friend, visit their acquaintance for a minimum of four hours a month to promote social, recreational, or educational activities.

Compeer has been recognized as a model mental health volunteer organization (The President's Service Award, three Points of Light awards). Dr. John McIntyre, a past president of the American Psychiatric Association, cites the group's greatest benefit as the degree of its contribution to the decreased stigma surrounding the public's perception of mental illness.

Compeer promotional materials inform readers how its programs—presently also engaging businesses and service organizations—can be supported at a much lower cost to taxpayers than the rehospitalization and homelessness circumstances of persons with mental illness can. Its statistics suggest how volunteer friendships tend to lower rehospitalization and suicide rates. And recent materials encourage applications for Robert Wood Johnson "Faith in Action" grants for fundraising, with religious congregations as chief sources for volunteer recruitment. Bernice Skirboll, executive director and founder, says that the quality necessary to be helpful is simply "*you* and your beliefs. It is what you're willing to share with another person."[6]

Julie has become a partner with Eunice, a Compeer volunteer. Here is what she has to say about the program:

> My Compeer friend and I have a mutual interest in movies and athletic sports. We have gone shopping, seen movies and taken car rides. . . . I am happy to discover that we both desire and strive for some common goals. These include self-respect, the joys of friendship, and a willingness to participate in the journeys of others who live with mental illnesses.[7]

For Christians, sharing one's beliefs and congregational commitments become a part of caring. The needs, let's remind ourselves, are complex; people coping with major mental illness encounter medical, social, housing, and financial demands. Congregational human resources are great, but caring cannot be left to good will and chance. To social events and continuing education opportunities add the potential Compeer contact. In them believers who care enough about mental health can become crucial advocates on practical levels.

Those of us who detect "involved" disciples in congregational life may also recall the Master's testimony: "By this everyone will know that you are my disciples, if you have love for one another" (John 13:35). Let me from a grateful heart share a few examples among so many others besides.

WHEN SHADOWS FADE

As the Apostle wrote to a Colossian friend so long ago, "the hearts of the saints have been refreshed through you" (Philem. 7). I likewise find encouragement from sharing the faith with others who with vision, initiative, and discipleship already have shown the courage to care.

Having recovered from a siege of depression, a clergy friend of mine mulled over an idea. Could he link the episode to professional ministry of a different kind? Could blessing arise from trial and despair? After seeking advice from folks at his local mental health center in Tacoma, Washington, a vision took hold: an ecumenical chaplaincy for chronic sufferers and their families.

Sponsorship emerged from a county interfaith ministries association. Acquiring support from this respected public religious agency became a heartening stimulus for further outreach. Next, a mental health chaplaincy board—recruited from consumers and family members—pledged support. Among its consumer family members, a physician, an attorney, and a college professor came aboard. They met for conversations, sensed the pastor's sincerity and confidence, and went to work.

At that time the name of the game was foundation grant monies. And, upon further resolve, perseverance, and prayer the "payoffs" began to arrive. There were not only grant awards. One congregation also joined in by offering a well-equipped office. Others provided meeting facilities and grants. Associated Ministries included project publicity in its newsletter, and a local Christian school gave Chaplain Paul part-time employment.

Today several area congregations schedule October Mental Health Sunday classes in adult Christian education programs. There are consumer support groups as well. A compeer program has its own director and continues to expand its contacts. The chaplain calls at board and care homes and teaches spiritual subjects—such as prayer, for instance—at day treatment programs in mental health centers. A new professional ministry has arisen; furthermore, the open door for an expanded ministry beckons.[8]

Then there are Susan and Gunnar Christiansen, parents of a son with schizophrenia and members of a large Presbyterian congregation in California. Gunnar has chaired the Religious Outreach committee of Orange County's Alliance for the Mentally Ill. In 1991 his committee distributed a questionnaire with reference to religious outreach to approximately 1,200 area churches. Seventeen responded; of these only a few reported any activity in this area. The only significant response was from a Lutheran pastor whose brother was ill with schizophrenia. Given such a response the committee decided that if anything was to be accomplished it would have to occur within their individual parishes rather than from the well-meaning efforts of their own committee.

So the Christiansens went to work engaging St. Andrew's Church of Newport Beach. Susan, during an adult Bible class late in 1993, asked for prayers on behalf of Chris, their son, who had just been committed to a mental institution for the second time. Her willingness to disclose such parental anxiety resulted in six ladies out of the forty-five in attendance coming to her to relate that they themselves or someone in their immediate family was suffering from mental illness. She had broken the ice for the subsequent adult education on the topic.

Gunnar decided to write the senior pastor a letter in the belief "that St. Andrew's might choose to accept new avenues in its religious outreach to those afflicted with chronic mental illness." Refining the context of the dream, he continued:

> Misunderstanding of the etiology and characteristics of schizophrenia, manic depression and chronic unipolar depression persists despite clarification by medical research. This lack of understanding has resulted in pervasive stigma which tends to cause those with mental illness to seek refuge in isolation. It is unfortunate that the reality we hope mentally ill patients with hallucinations will regain is at present a reality which includes the repressive force of this stigma.
>
> By following the direction set by Christ in attending the needs of the mentally ill, the Church has the potential of having a significant positive impact on the views of society.[9]

Upon gaining their clergy's support, the Christiansens organized a task force for follow-up efforts and spoke before various groups to complement congregational adult education initiatives. A highlight of 1996 was an all-day conference held at St. Andrew's for clergy and lay leaders of churches and synagogues in the Orange County area. The "Hope and Help for Serious Mental Illness" affair drew 300 participants, 250 of them from other faith communities. During the sessions competent experts supervised several workshops. A harvest from seeds of steady, intentional discipleship had begun, as people took home with them a new challenge (Rom. 1:13).[10]

From small beginnings seventeen years ago, "Faith and Fellowship" is a parish-based program of small-group faith sharing. This plan is tailored to meet the unique needs of persons with severe and persistent mental illness living outside the hospital setting. Three groups minister today in Chicago/Oak Park and two in Saginaw, Michigan. Empathy from "healthy" and "normal" folks can do much to break the pain and isolation of those whose psychiatric and social situations lead to fragile faith and self-esteem ("Do I look and act okay here?"). For some, regular church-going becomes not a place of hope but a place of risk. A rejecting community may suggest a rejecting God. Depression lurks. A faith and fellowship group, however, can become "church" for shy and anxious inquirers. Their presence, they learn, is not just tolerated; it is sought and cherished.[11]

Contemplate the action of a similar group, "Second MILERS," at First United Methodist in Tulsa, Oklahoma. The acronym MILE (*M*ental *I*llness, a *L*oving *E*mbrace) writes Barbara Schneeberg, came "after a search for words that captured our dream of offering more than a touch."[12] Second MILE partners with a public agency: Mobile Outreach Crisis Services. When a team of Tulsa mental health professionals routinely sweep neighborhoods in search of those willing and able to come in off the streets it goes into action. Trained church care teams then befriend these *formerly* homeless ones during the critical transition period. "We see a rainbow of promise arching over a desolate trail," adds Barbara. "Soon the term 'client' converted in our hearts to 'person' and then 'friend.'"[13]

We have given the nod to models of ministry *to* and *with* the persistently mentally ill and their families. Let's turn the page in search of ministry *by* them.

Chapter 8

Habits of Presence

The cup of blessing that we bless, is it not a sharing in the blood of Christ?

1 Cor. 10:16

Faith and love are timeless acts which remove us out of time, because they make us wholly present.

Jürgen Moltmann
Theology of Hope

Hospital quarters, group home hallways, and stained glass sanctuaries all provide noteworthy settings for psychiatric disability caring. As efforts continue for months and years, however, caregivers may also perceive a call for their attentions in the long run. Failing independent living arrangements and rehospitalization events invite a surrender to the long-term, persistent, chronic illness. For everyone, submission to it will entail a test of priority setting and will.

Consider the challenge through the eyes of the father of David, a thirty-something man diagnosed with paranoid schizophrenia:

> Of foremost importance in giving care to families of the mentally ill is the minister's own attitude toward mental illness. The question must be asked, "Are these people and their families my responsibility?" They usually require long-term care and there are often crisis situations which can be confusing and even frightening. This can require much energy, time and patience—qualities that a busy pastor may be unwilling to give. This price must be given serious consideration.[1]

There are shepherds of the flock (1 Peter 5:3) who will nonetheless forsake indifference and become examples of caring ministry by their intentional "yes" to the disturbing question of responsibility. To support their resolve in long-range consent, I post two maintenance standards:

ALLIES AND FRIENDS

Research suggests that while families with a mentally ill member highly value pastoral visitation, a caring attitude, prayer, and counseling from their pastor, they would most like him or her to mobilize a caring ministry among members of the congregation.[2]

From the secular viewpoint, researchers have concluded that although the psychological and social approach to understanding physical disability has a long tradition, such is not the case with psychiatric disability. Here the traditional emphasis has been upon treating the illness rather than the person who has the illness. Further, it has neither acknowledged the impact of the helping system and society in general on the person struggling to recover nor recognized the impact on families. Today, however, they cite a gradual change toward "language that is more respectful of, and consistent with, how people with psychiatric disability view themselves."[3]

Amidst the language of *praxis* and *treatment*, the voice of theology will contribute a distinctive tone: "Now faith, hope, and love abide, these three; and the greatest of these is love" (1 Cor. 13:13). As bearers of this message, pastors are not called to explain things but rather to bear witness to truth, the pain of the person, and the hope found in God's ultimate promises. These include confessing to the realities of life's limitations, to suffering, and ultimately to the mystery of dying.

Our culture's entertainment and "success" agenda is aimed at distracting us from the truth of what it means to be human in a sinful world. Suffering is or will be present. Jesus confronted struggle in Gethsemane (Mark 14:32-42). Suffering, such as that surrounding mental illness, contradicts our sense of the way the world should be. But Gethsemane and the Cross are followed by Easter and Resurrection. "God-talk" is thus both a pastor's privilege and responsibility. It also involves the overseer (ombudsman) prophet-like role.

To illustrate, consider how Lewis L. Judd, MD, of the National Institute of Mental Health exposes commonly held myths.[4]

Myth 1: Mental disorders are not as "real" as other illnesses. New scientific technology permits researchers to see structure and activity in living human brains. There is graphic evidence that severe mental illnesses are connected to demonstrable brain dysfunction. Myth 1 contributes to political decisions made by officials. For example, while federal funds for the National Institute of Health (NIH) have been increased by 35 to 40 percent over the past twenty years, National Institute for Mental Health (NIMH) funding decreased by 14 percent during the same period.

Myth 2: By comparison to other illnesses mental disorders are uncommon. Schizophrenia is five times more common than multiple sclerosis, six times more common than insulin-dependent diabetes, and sixty times more widespread than muscular dystrophy. One in five Americans will have a mental disability at some time in life.

Myth 3: Those suffering from mental disorders are adequately served by medical practitioners and public institutions. In fact, only one-fifth of adults with mental disorders of any type are receiving care; furthermore, they suffer from discriminatory health insurance practices. In the field of medicine Dr. Judd reports that psychiatry has become virtually the only specialty experiencing a shortage of practitioners.[5]

Into this scene steps the pastor. With continuing "leading learner" efforts (Chapter 6), he or she could speak out in church and elsewhere to help counter the falsehoods cited on Dr. Judd's list. But let's pose the leading question once more. Are persons with mental disorders and their families a minister's responsibility? When the messes encountered in parishioners' lives seem so much greater than the resources available to solve them, the pastor could murmur, "I guess not." Besides, anyone can become anxious that stress overload could simply overwhelm the earnest, well-intentioned caregiver. We resign ourselves to powerlessness. Like ancient Israel, we can taste the bitter waters of exile (Psalm 137:1).

I insist, however, that no matter how little mental health expertise or skills clergy may think they have to offer, none must let themselves be blinded to the one helpful action always at hand. Pastors can become allies to families in sorrow. They can show compassion. Instead of worrying about what to say they can stop and simply try to *listen*. Sister Helen Prejean's *Dead Man Walking*, made into a film starring Susan Sarandon and Sean Penn, illustrates this powerless presence of identifying with our crucified but risen Lord.

In such ministry, *being* comes before doing or telling. It means adopting a form of servanthood characterized by suffering alongside of and with the hurt; it will take seriously a hidden discipline behind public proclamations and celebrations. Grounded in the doctrine of Christ's Incarnation, it recalls the Lord "who emptied himself, taking the form of a servant" (Phil. 2:7-8). Spiritual growth and empowerment will look at the servant's cross for inspiration in plans to fuse presence with action.[6] A loving God can comfort even in the face of madness in the family.

A sense of the experience of power or "presence" seems to undergird all religion. Among the ancient Hebrews Yahweh manifests sacred being in habitations such as the cloud and the "glory" (Hebrew *cabod*) filling the Tabernacle (Exod. 40:34). Presence is also mediated in processes connected to *fertility* or recurring *seasons*, in *events* such as the birth of Jesus, or in *special places* at shrines and temples.[7] It also appears in *persons* such as Moses. In the fourth Gospel, John claims that Jesus "the Word" became flesh (Greek "pitch a tent") and the disciples see his "glory" (Greek *doxa*, John 1:14). In *special communities*—Israel as a Chosen People and the Church as the Body of Christ—a story of tensions resulting from God's felt presence or abandonment unfolds.

Its plot could never unfold apart from prophets such as Ezekiel, Amos, Jeremiah, and all the rest. "The prophet," writes Abraham Heschel, "was an individual who said no to his society, condemning its habits and assumptions, its complacency . . ."[8] Although the scholar notes what happened *to* prophets, he rather emphasizes what happened *in* them. Pathos (from Latin *pati*, to suffer) would emerge as the basic feature in the seer's consciousness. The prophetic attitude embraced sympathy both *with* God and *for* God.[9]

> I gave you cleanness of teeth in all your cities,
> and lack of bread in all your places,
> yet you did not return to me, says the Lord. . .
> Seek good and not evil, that you may live;
> and so the Lord, the God of hosts will be with you,
> just as you have said. (Amos 4:6, 5:14)

The quickest association we tend to make with the word prophet today is predicting the future. But prior to future pronouncements, their inner suffering breaks out to condemn the fallout from evil habits in place among their fellow citizenry:

> For scoundrels are found among my people . . .
> They know no limits in deeds of wickedness;
> they do not judge with justice
> the cause of the orphan, to make it prosper,
> and they do not defend the rights of the needy. (Jer. 5:26-28)

Substitute the deinstitutionalized homeless mentally ill for "orphan" and criminalizing the hallucinating victim for the "rights of the needy." Recall the ridicule and the humiliation of families portrayed in previous chapters and the prophetic call echoes still.

Prophecy extends to New Testament times as well. In the early Church it appears among those who felt a call or gift for inspired utterance (1 Cor. 14:1, 37). Their ministry might have been conducted singly, in groups or within a given congregation. Sometimes it extended throughout a region (Acts 15:22, 32-36; 21:10-11). These gifted ones also were associated with teachers of the Church at Antioch (Acts 13:1).[10] I claim that "inspired utterance" today belongs not so much to political analysis or fearsome predictions about the future as to the cultivation of empathic insights reflected in ordinary preaching and teaching times. It means becoming an up-to-date ally of the truths about mental illness.

It is easy to overlook the prophets' inner life because we are so accustomed to their jeremiads and bold accusations:

> Thus says the Lord:
> For three transgressions of Damascus and for four,

I will not revoke the punishment . . .
Hear this word, you cows of Bashan
who are on Mount Samaria,
who oppress the poor,
who crush the needy,
who say to their husbands, "Bring something to drink!" (Amos
1:3, 4:1)

In New Testament times, however, James the brother of Jesus recalls something else:

As an example of suffering and patience, beloved, take
the prophets who spoke in the name of the Lord. (James 5:10)

Isaiah of Jerusalem illustrates patient suffering. He senses the failure of his previous teaching and confrontation but will not give in to cynicism and despair.

Bind up the testimony,
seal the teaching among my disciples.
I will wait for the Lord,
who is hiding his face from the house of Jacob,
and I will hope in Him. (Isa. 8:16-17) (NKJV)

Given a seemingly absent God the religious presence of the eighth-century Judean prophet and his family will remain in Jerusalem (Isa. 8:18).

Up to this point, I have been urging public pastoral concern for families bearing burdens of mental illness. Yet so often clergy care-giving will seem only to have begun after the acute-stage crisis. As signs of cure seem to fade old challenges appear in more hidden ways. Yet families and their professional care collaborators will still hang on.

Clergy who care will emulate the hope of Isaiah's wait by daring to represent a prophetic challenge to "harmonial" (avoiding para-dox and suffering) religion. Allies of affected families, they will also become advocates with them.

PROMOTING HOPE

Becoming allies and friends of families coping with brain disorders guides my first habit of presence. *Belief* joins the second recommended habit. A professor of pastoral care provides content for such context when he writes:

> The pastor does not have knowledge of ultimate realities to which other humans are not privy. But the pastor knows that it makes a difference—a practical difference—whether one believes or not, and knows that the difference is captured in this modest and unassuming word "hope."[11]

He contends that pastors are primarily providers or agents of hope. These managers may endure frustration in acting out a gatekeeper role and will respect balance in personal engagements.

Major threats to a hopeful attitude toward life are despair, apathy, and shame. In contrast, major supports for a hopeful attitude are trust, patience, and modesty. The ultimate experience lies in the future, that is, in our own death when we relinquish our hold on this life and entrust it to God.[12]

Endurance

In time the sense of loss and grieving resurfaces. As one spouse of an Alzheimer's casualty put it, "All you have is a shell, mocking what once was." Public outpourings of sympathetic actions will comfort grieving parents, spouses, and siblings after unexpected and tragic events. However, mental disorders and Alzheimer's cases will produce something different, a "disenfranchised" grief, since observers hardly know what to think or do. So the ache remains undercover and some sufferers cannot seem to "mourn decently."[13]

Ambivalent feelings surround the situation. Parents may still think if they had acted upon those early signs of disorders things might have gone differently. Hidden refrains of guilt peal on: "If only we had acted sooner . . . if only I had tried to be a more understanding spouse . . . if only I had paid attention."

Anger stirs up resentments for the postures of relatives and friends that are perceived as unsympathetic. Society itself, considered to be wallowing in stereotyping and hypocrisy, must share responsibility. Little wonder, then, that the health care system failed them, family copers bitterly conclude. Kept in secrecy and shame, such attitudes fester and demoralize. In the minds of some a grudging impatience even questions whether the sufferer has actually lost all control over the recovery process; maybe the so-called victims are partly to blame.[14]

For ministry such ambiguity cries out for "fruit of the Spirit . . . love, peace, kindness, self-control . . . patience" (Gal. 5:22-23). In contrast to the classical use of the Greek word for patience, William Barclay cites its characteristically Christian interpretations: (1) it defines "a steadfast spirit which never gives in," and (2) the attitude one can display toward others, an ideal goal for every minister and church member. The groundwork for all this, he concludes, is God's own patience with us.[15]

Gatekeeper

A hidden discipline of endurance is not an end in itself. Any pastor who combines perception and empathy with such family stresses will also want to make his or her presence felt in practical ways.

First of all, conversation, structured or informal, will seek to label the ambiguities of care and feelings. Questions such as, "If God loves us so much, why do we suffer this way?" and, Is God punishing us?" can open access to Bible texts such as Job and to the struggle of Gethsemane. By honest questioning we can express frustrations and join the fellowship of others who share the pain. Harold Kushner's book, *When Bad Things Happen to Good People*[16] and the film about C. S. Lewis, *Shadowlands,* provide stimulating and open-minded insights. Resources of prayer and Bible text can console, help searchers accept the situation as it actually exists and, in trust, commit the future to hope in God's promises.

The second opportunity for ministry takes into account an extended family circle. A pastor may be key to organizing conversations with several generations present. Shared perceptions of crises and needs may become a base for a teamwork response to provide respite time in sharing the load. Emerging from such discussions, family rituals for holidays and anniversaries can be adapted rather than abandoned. The same holds true for birthdays. There is life, even amidst ambiguous loss.[17]

Third, an opening for support concerns the ongoing need for information. Telephone numbers for the local mental health center, National Alliance for the Mentally Ill offices, and recommended counselors may require updating. Investigate respite care possibilities in the congregation. Encouragement of a "take charge" versus a "reacting as best we can" attitude will minimize feelings of entrapment and helplessness.

Pastors are not magicians but connecting defeated family members with any of the above options can work wonders. Even a telephone inquiry can offset severe isolation and, for some, represent the presence of the living Christ.

Balance

The foregoing pages of this chapter have discussed how clergy can minister to the family burden of mental illness by sharing the load with their presence. I underscore next a necessity for safeguarding such ministry in the face of sometimes tiresome chronic outcomes and dashed rehabilitation hopes. This means, first of all, that keeping a personal balance, or stress management, must not be left to chance.

Medical doctors use a system of being "on call" to maintain coverage for medical treatment and emergencies. It guarantees their long-term stress situations will be shared by other professionals. Overall the system has gained broad public acceptance. In contrast, professional clergy are frequently locked into an unwritten church expectation that they will be on call twenty-four hours a day, seven days a week.

Caught amid a myriad of activities in Galilee, Jesus counsels his disciples, "Come away and rest awhile" (Mark 6:30-31). Sometimes people with chronic mental illnesses appear to orchestrate their various caregiver benefactors in a crescendo of service deadlines. Family members are placed on call as are health care people; so also social workers and, at times, educators and counselors as well. Pastors, too, can become caught up in the swing of things. Sharing the burden, however, has a boundary line of obligation each caregiver will have to decide upon. Clergy need to sharpen insights—by experience and advice from such colleagues—about separating emergency distress signals from chronic ones. "Come away and rest awhile." Even the Master says so. And this applies not only to parishioner needs but also to a pastor's private and family life.

C. Welton Gaddy, a prominent Baptist minister, received psychiatric hospitalization. He writes about it in *A Soul Under Siege* and offers a fascinating description of the onset of clinical depression together with practical advice about dangers inherent in playing God for the congregation.[18]

As we have seen, families bearing mental illness burdens endure shattered dreams and nonclosure grief. Yet so far as "church" is concerned they look not so much for pastoral heroes or faith cures as for emissaries who simply acknowledge the pain. Such gestures help much more than what seems to be perpetual avoidance for fear of embarrassment.

The Rivers family (see Chapter 4) and the situation with Randy's bipolar illness brings home the point. Back in times when Randy was fairly active in the church youth group, Julie Jones was also part of the gang going to youth conventions. Not long afterward, Julie learned she had been admitted to an Ivy League university, a first for the congregation. And Pastor Perry took note enough to visit the Jones family. Upon sharing their joy he went on to ask Julie for feedback about life at Harvard. He also predicted challenges to her faith. Nevertheless he assured her of their confidence she might even benefit from them; she was now off on her own but their prayers would follow after. He was optimistic she would continue to make them all proud in her preparation for service to others. The hidden benefit resulting from pastoral care for an achiever such as Julie countered his sad concern for "nonachievers" such as Randy.

CONSUMERS OF CAREGIVING:
THEIR PRESENCE

Julie was poised to leave home. Having grown spiritually and intellectually, her future radiated promise. Not so with Randy. No new stage of growth or independence appeared in the offing. This parishioner's struggle to fit in went on, and Pastor Perry determined at least to keep in touch with the family.

In terms of future contacts the pastor could anticipate "ministry *with*" Julie; in Randy's case, however, should there be contact at all, it would be on a "ministry *to*" basis. Or would it? A leading British churchman writes:

> The poor, the deprived, the handicapped are not primarily a problem to be solved by the rich, the comfortable and the strong. They are the bearers of a witness without which the strong are lost in their own illusions. They are the trustees of a blessing without which the church cannot bless the world.
>
> Their presence in the church is the indispensable correction of our inveterate tendency to identify the power of God with our power, the victory of God with our success. Because they keep us close to the reality of the cross, they can bring to us also, if we are willing to see, the light of a new day which dawns from beyond our horizons and which is close to us in the resurrection of the crucified.[19]

Those who risk becoming present with such witnesses among us may discover realities of the mysterious blessings they have offered to so many. Simple joys, modest ambition, and generosity mark its evidence. Every caregiver can provide a story of "ministry *from*" these negated neighbors, perhaps the very ones to be amazed by fulfillment of the Lord's promise, "But many who are first will be last, and the last will be first" (Matt. 19:30).

In his book *Meeting Jesus Again for the First Time*, Marcus Borg describes three "macro-stories" of Scripture that shape the Bible as a whole. Each of them images religious life in a particular way. The first one relates the narrative of the exodus from Egypt. Found here are themes of liberation from bondage plus the journey stretching toward a far-off destination. An account of the exile and return from Babylon follows. Powerlessness and marginality will become a part of Israel's memory ever afterwards. The final macro-story takes place not so much in the history of ancient Israel as in the life of its institutions—the temple in Jerusalem, the priesthood, and sacrifice. Religious life now connects to worship and heartfelt obedience to the Deity and Torah as reflected in the pathos and pleas of the prophets.[20]

Micro-stories in our lives seem to parallel the unfolding drama of Israel's past. They describe how through medication and psychotherapy individuals burdened with schizophrenia and depression can find themselves liberated enough to leave the hospital. Yet failures with medication plans initiate relapse. Powerless and homeless, the exiles then learn once more about life on the margins of acceptance by Newbigin's "the rich, the comfortable, and the strong." Sooner or later a quest for housing, rehabilitation, and social life will engage institutions of the health care system. New identities of both sufferers and caregivers arise along the way. All three of the great stories seem to blend together in time and exposure.

The living God has promised a Presence to both community and individual and promises that an onslaught of present sufferings will not prevail (Rom. 8:18). Retelling the stories—big and small, old and new—will support us as we open our lives to a ministry of presence.

Appendix

Sources for Information

DENOMINATION NETWORKS

Pastor Lisa T. Clever
Director for Disability Ministries
Division for Church and Society
Evangelical Lutheran Church in America
8765 West Higgins Road
Chicago, IL 60631-4190
(800) 638-3522 ext. 2692

Annette Stixrud, Executive Director
Northwest Parish Nurse Ministries
2801 N. Gantebein Ave., Room 1072
Portland, OR 97227
FAX (503) 413-2407

Florence Kraft
Chair, Presbyterian Serious Mental Illness Network
1151 - 48th Ave. #107
Chula Vista, CA 91911
(619) 422-2733

INTERFAITH

Jennifer Shifrin, Executive Director
Pathways to Promise
131 West Monroe, Suite 8
St. Louis, MO 63122

SECULAR ORGANIZATIONS

The National Alliance for the Mentally Ill (NAMI) has literature for siblings, offspring, parents, other relatives, and friends, as well as consumers. NAMI has chapters in all fifty states. To locate a group in your area, or to obtain information regarding starting either a Siblings and Adult Children or Spouses and Partners support group, call or write to NAMI's national headquarters:

> National Alliance for the Mentally Ill
> 200 North Glebe Road, Suite 1015
> Arlington, VA 22203-3754
> (703) 524-7600; Fax (703) 524-9094
> toll-free 1-800-950-NAMI

The National Depressive and Manic-Depressive Association, for consumers and their families, has chapters in most states. Call or write to the organization's national headquarters:

> National Depressive and Manic-Depressive Association
> 730 North Franklin Street, Suite 501
> Chicago, IL 60610-3526
> (312) 642-0049; Fax (312) 642-7243
> toll-free 1-800-82-NDMDA

Siblings of people with disabilities can get literature and information from the following sources:

> Siblings for Significant Change
> United Charities Building
> 105 East 22nd Street
> New York, NY 10010
> (212) 420-0776

> Sibling Support Project
> Children's Hospital & Medical Center
> 4800 Sand Point Way N.E.
> P.O. Box 5371
> Seattle, WA 98105-0371
> (206) 368-4911; Fax (206) 368-4816

Sibling Information Network
The University of Connecticut
A.J. Pappanikou Center
249 Glenbrook Road, U-64
Storrs, CT 06269-2064
(203) 486-4985

The National Institute of Mental Health (NIMH) publishes a variety of pamphlets about various brain disorders. These publications, available at the addresses listed below, describe the symptoms, causes, and treatments, and are free.

For information about depression, NIMH has developed a public education program called D/ART (an acronym for Depression Awareness, Recognition, and Treatment). Call or write to:

D/ART, NIMH
5600 Fisher Lane, Room 10-85
Rockville, MD 20857
(301) 443-4140
For a free brochure call 1-800-421-4211

A public company dedicated to serving the Seriously Mentally Ill (SMI) population:

PMR Corporation
501 Washington Street
San Diego, CA 92103
(619) 610-4074; Fax (619) 610-4184

For information about schizophrenia, write:

Public Inquiries Branch
National Institute of Mental Health
Room 15C-05
5600 Fisher Lane
Rockville, MD 20857

American Psychiatric Association
1400 K Street N.W.
Washington, DC 20005
(202) 682-6220

Center for Psychiatric Rehabilitation
Boston University
930 Commonwealth Avenue
Boston, MA 02215
(617) 353-3549

PRIMARY RESOURCES

Reference Works

Dictionary of Pastoral Care and Counseling (R. Hunter, Liston O. Mills, and John Patton, eds.), many helpful articles such as "Mental Health and Illness," "Psychopathology, Theories of"; note especially "Schizophrenia," pp. 1116-1119.
Encyclopedia Judaica, Vol. II, "Mental Illness," pp. 1374-1378.
Encyclopedia of Religion (Mircea Eliade, ed.), Vol. IV, "Demons," pp. 288-292; Vol. XII, "Psychology and Religion Movement," pp. 66-75; "Psychotherapy and Religion," pp. 75-80.
The Mennonite Encyclopedia, Vol. III, "Mental Hospitals, Mennonite," pp. 653-654.
New Catholic Encyclopedia, Vol. IX, "Mental Health," pp. 658-660.
Theological Word Book of the New Testament (G. Kittel, ed.), Vol. IV, "mad"; "madness" pp. 360-361, 962-963.

Books

American Psychiatric Association, *Let's Talk Facts About Schizophrenia*, Washington, DC: APA, 1988.
American Psychiatric Association, *A Mental Illness Awareness Guide for Clergy*, Washington, DC: APA, 1990.
Robert H. Albers, *Shame: A Faith Perspective*, Binghamton, NY: The Haworth Press, 1995.

Nancy C. Andreason, *The Broken Brain: The Biological Revolution in Psychiatry*, New York: Harper and Row, 1984.

William Anthony, Mikal Cohen, Marianne Farkas, *Psychiatric Rehabilitation*, Boston: Center for Psychiatric Rehabilitation, 1990.

Donald Capps, *Agents of Hope: A Pastoral Psychology* (Minneapolis, MN: Fortress Press, 1995).

Anne Deveson, *Tell Me I'm Here*. Victoria, Australia: Penguin, 1991.

J. Moltmann, *The Way of Jesus Christ* (Minneapolis, MN: Fortress Press, 1990).

Carol North, *Welcome Silence: My Triumph Over Schizophrenia*, New York: Simon and Schuster, 1987.

A. Preheim-Bartel, Aldred H. Neufeldt, *Supportive Care in the Congregation* (Akron, PA: Mennonite Central Committee, 1986).

E. Fuller Torrey, *Surviving Schizophrenia—A Family Manual*, Third edition New York: Harper and Row, 1995.

E. Fuller Torrey, *Nowhere to Go: The Tragic Odyssey of the Homeless Mentally Ill*, New York: Harper and Row, 1988.

Otto F. Wahl, *Media Madness: Public Images of Mental Illness*, New Brunswick, NJ: Rutgers University Press, 1995.

Selected Articles

Clark S. Aist, "Pastoral Care of the Mentally Ill," *The Journal of Pastoral Care* (December 1987), pp. 299-310.

John M. Cannon, "Pastoral Care for Families of the Mentally Ill," *The Journal of Pastoral Care* (Fall 1990), pp. 213-221.

Rosalynn Carter, "A Voice for the Voiceless: The Church and the Mentally Ill," *Second Opinion* (Vol. 13 1990), pp. 44-48.

H. Paul Chalfant, Peter Heller, Alden Roberts, David Briones, Salvador Aguirre-Hochbaum, Walter Farr, "The Clergy as Resource for Those Encountering Psychological Distress," *Review of Religious Research* (March, 1990), pp. 305-313.

H.T. Engelhardt, "The Social Meanings of Illness," *Second Opinion* (Vol. 1 1986), pp. 26-39.

Richard C. Erickson, David Cutler, Victoria Cowell, and George Dobler, "Serving the Needs of Persons with Chronic Mental

Illness: A Neglected Ministry." *The Journal of Pastoral Care* (Summer, 1990), pp. 153-162.

Florence Kraft, "The Church and Serious Mental Illness," *Church and Society* (January/February 1991). Presbyterian Serious Mental Illness Network, pp. 2-5.

Robert Michals, "Psychiatry: Where Medicine, Psychology and Ethics Meet," *Second Opinion,* Vol. 6, 1987, 35-48.

Andrew J. Weaver, "Has There Been a Failure to Prepare and Support Parish-Based Clergy in Their Role as Frontline Community Mental Health Workers: A Review," *Church and Society* (Summer, 1995), pp. 129-147.

James P. Wind, "A Place for Madness?" *Second Opinion,* Vol. 3, 1986, 52-90.

Word and World (Spring 1989) The entire issue is devoted to the subject of ministry and mental health. Biblical, theological, and personal accounts.

The Family and Mental Illness

Elizabeth Achtemeier, *Preaching About Family Relationships* (Philadelphia: The Westminster Press, 1987).

Patricia Backlar, *The Family Face of Schizophrenia* (New York: Putnam, 1994).

George Bennett, *When the Mental Patient Comes Home* (Philadelphia: The Westminster Press, 1980).

H. Paul Chalfant, Peter Heller, Alden Roberts, David Briones, Salvador Aguirre-Hochbaum, Walter Farr, "The Clergy as a Resource for Those Encountering Psychological Distress," *Review of Religious Research* (March 1990), pp. 305-312.

The Experiences of Patients and Families: First Person Accounts (Arlington, VA: National Alliance for the Mentally Ill, 1989).

Erica E. Goode, *U.S. News and World Report* "When Mental Illness Hits Home"(April 24, 1989), pp. 54-65.

Agnes B. Hatfield, Leroy Spaniol, and Anthony M. Zipple, "Expressed Emotion: A Family Perspective," *Schizophrenia Bulletin* 1(2), 221-225.

Margaret O. Hyde, *Is This Kid Crazy?* (Philadelphia: The Westminster Press, 1983).

Liz Kuipers, Julian Leff, Dominic Lam, *Family Work for Schizophrenia: A Practical Guide* (London: Gaskell, 1992).

Harriet P. Lefley and Dale L. Johnson (eds.), *Families as Allies in the Treatment of the Mentally Ill: New Directions for Mental Health Professionals* (Washington, DC: American Psychiatric Press, 1990).

Arthur C. McGill, *Suffering: A Test of Theological Method* (Philadelphia: The Westminster Press, 1982).

Kim T. Mueser and Susan Gingerich, *Coping with Schizophrenia: A Guide for Families* (Oakland, CA: New Harbinger Publications, 1994).

Victoria Secunda, *When Madness Comes Home: Help and Hope for the Children, Siblings, and Partners of the Mentally Ill* (New York: Hyperion, 1997).

Jennifer Shifrin, Jeffrey Cohen, Florence Kraft (eds.), *Pathways to Partnership: An Awareness and Research Guide on Mental Illness* (St. Louis, MO: Pathways to Promise, 1997).

Clea Simon, *Mad House* (New York: Doubleday, 1997).

Shirley G. Strobel, *Creating a Circle of Caring: The Church and the Mentally Ill* (Raleigh, NC: North Carolina Alliance for the Mentally Ill, 1997).

Colleen Syalor, "The Management of Stigma," *Holistic Nursing Practice* (October 1990), 45-53.

William L. Vaswig, *I Prayed, He Answered* (Minneapolis: Augsburg Publishing House, 1980).

Phyllis Vine, *Families in Pain: Children, Siblings, Spouses, and Parents of the Mentally Ill Speak Out* (New York: Pantheon Books, 1982).

Mona Wasow, *The Skipping Stone: Ripple Effects of Mental Illness on the Family* (Palo Alto, CA: Science and Behavior Books, 1995).

Rebecca Woolis, *When Someone You Love Has a Mental Illness: A Handbook for Family, Friends, and Caregivers* (New York: G.P. Putnam's Sons, 1992).

Films and Documentaries

Man Facing Southeast (Argentina), Dallas Pictures, New World Video, 1987.

One Flew Over the Cuckoo's Nest, 1975

Alfred Hitchcock, *Psycho*, 1960

Through a Glass Darkly (Sweden), Janus Films, Embassy Home
    Entertainment, 1961

The Brain (series), (PBS)

"The Broken Mind" (*Frontline*, 1990) (PBS)

Shine (Australia), 1996

"News from Medicine Presents: Peace of Mind," CNN. 1992.
    Public Relations Department, NAMI, Arlington, VA 22209

Crazy People, 1990

The Silence of the Lambs, 1992

Notes

Introduction

1. E. Fuller Torrey, *Surviving Schizophrenia: A Manual for Families, Consumers and Providers*, Third edition (New York: Harper Collins, 1995), 21-24.

2. Clea Simon, *Mad House: Growing up in the Shadow of Mentally Ill Siblings* (New York: Doubleday, 1997).

3. Iris V. Cully and Kendig B. Cully (gen. eds.) *Harper's Encyclopedia of Religious Education* (San Francisco: Harper and Row, 1990), 98-103.

4. Diane T. Marsh and Rex M. Dickens, *Troubled Journey: Coming to Terms with the Mental Illness of a Sibling or Parent* (New York: Penguin Putnam, Inc., 1997), 25.

5. Stewart Govig, *Souls Are Made of Endurance: Surviving Mental Illness in the Family* (Louisville: Westminster John Knox Press, 1994).

6. Jürgen Moltmann, *The Coming of God* (Minneapolis: Fortress Press, 1996), 267. See Psalms 95:2 and 139.

7. Unless otherwise noted, all Bible quotations are taken from the New Revised Standard Version (NRSV) (New York: Oxford University Press, 1991).

8. Gunnar E. Christiansen, in Jennifer Shifrin (ed.) *Caring Congregations: Observations and Commentary* (St. Louis, MO: Pathways to Promise, 1997), 39.

9. Victoria Secunda, *When Madness Comes Home: Help and Hope for the Children, Siblings, and Partners of the Mentally Ill* (New York: Hyperion, 1997).

10. Diane T. Marsh and Rex M. Dickens, *Troubled Journey: Coming to Terms with the Mental Illness of Sibling or Parent* (New York: Penguin Putnam, Inc., 1997), 119.

11. LeRoy Spaniol, Cheryl Gagne, and Martin Koehler (eds.), *Psychological and Social Aspects of Psychiatric Disability* (Boston: Center for Psychiatric Rehabilitation, Boston University, 1997), pp. 156-171.

12. Harriet Lefley, *Family Caregiving in Mental Illness* (Thousand Oaks, CA: Sage Publications, 1996).

Chapter 1

1. Mark A. Winter, "Individuals with Serious Mental Illness: A Ministry Based on the Concept of Community" (DMin diss, San Francisco Theological Seminary, 1993), 1.

2. C.S. Aist, "Mental Health and Illness," *Dictionary of Pastoral Care and Counseling*, ed. Rodney J. Hunter (Nashville: Abingdon Press, 1990), 711.

3. Ruth C. Ackerman, *Twists and Turns: A Mother's Caring Journey* (Honeoye Falls, NY: Paths O Life Press, 1993), 142.

4. Carol North, *Welcome Silence: My Triumph Over Schizophrenia* (New York: Simon and Schuster, 1987), 60, 62.

5. E. Fuller Torrey, *Surviving Schizophrenia: A Manual for Families, Consumers and Providers*, Third edition (New York: Harper Collins, 1995), 58-60.

6. C. Welton Gaddy, *A Soul Under Siege: Surviving Clergy Depression* (Louisville, KY: Westminster John Knox Press, 1991), 17-21.

7. Torrey, *Surviving Schizophrenia*, 30. See Chapter 2 for further description and illustrations from case studies.

8. Arthur Frank, *At the Will of the Body: Reflections on Illness* (Boston: Houghton Mifflin Company, 1991), 12-13.

9. Torrey, *Surviving Schizophrenia*, 180.

10. Nancy C. Andreasen, *The Broken Brain* (New York: Harper and Row, 1984), 34-82. See also Torrey, *Surviving Schizophrenia*, Chapters 3 and 7.

11. Rebecca Woolis, *When Someone You Love Has a Mental Illness* (New York: G.P. Putnam's Sons, 1992), 23-34; National Alliance for the Mentally Ill (NAMI), *Understanding Schizophrenia* (Arlington, VA: n.d.), 5.

12. LeRoy Spaniol and Anthony M. Zipple, "The Family Recovery Process," *Psychological and Social Aspects of Psychiatric Disability*, ed. LeRoy Spaniol, Cheryl Gagne, and Martin Koehler (Boston: Boston University, 1997), 283.

13. William Anthony, Mikal Cohen, and Marianne Farkas, *Psychiatric Rehabilitation* (Boston: Center for Psychiatric Rehabilitation, 1990), 2.

14. Madelaine L'Engle, quoted in newsletter *Context*, Martin E. Marty, ed. Chicago: 24(13), 2.

15. Arthur Kleinman, *The Illness Narrative: Suffering, Healing, and the Human Condition* (New York: Basic Books, 1988), 108-109.

16. Jennifer Shifrin (ed.), Publication No. 86-1407. *Mental Illness Curriculum* (St. Louis: Pathways to Promise, 1994), 81.

17. Otto F. Wahl, *Media Madness: Public Images of Mental Illness* (New Brunswick, NJ: Rutgers University Press, 1995), 6-8.

18. Torrey, *Surviving Schizophrenia*, 2, 269-70.

19. *International Encyclopedia of the Social Sciences*, 1968 ed., "Pollution."

20. Winter, "Individuals with Serious Mental Illness," 39-41.

21. Daniel Migliore, "Mission in a Violent World," *The Princeton Seminary Bulletin* 17(1) (1996), 71-77.

Chapter 2

1. Mona Wasaw, *The Skipping Stone: Ripple Effects of Mental Illness on the Family* (Palo Alto, CA: Science and Behavior Books, 1995), 1, 205.

2. Anne Deveson, *Tell Me I'm Here* (Victoria, Australia: Penguin Books, 1991), 16.

3. Phyllis Vine, *Families in Pain: Children, Siblings, Spouses, and Parents of the Mentally Ill Speak Out* (New York: Pantheon Books, 1982), 12-21.

4. Groups for the Advancement of Psychiatry, *A Family Affair: Helping Families Cope with Mental Illness* (New York: Brunner/Mazel Publishers, 1986), 19-20.

5. Deveson, *Tell Me I'm Here*, 171-172.

6. Patricia Backlar, *The Family Face of Schizophrenia: Practical Counsel from America's Leading Experts* (New York: G.P. Putnam's Sons, 1994), 173.

7. Lisa Miller, "Surge in Malpractice Suits Leads Pastors to Offer Less Counseling to Parishioners." *The Wall Street Journal*, February 5, 1998, B1, 13.

8. Gerald F. Hawthorne, "Peace," in Bruce M. Metzger and Michael D. Coogan (eds.), *The Oxford Companion to the Bible* (New York: Oxford University Press, 1993), 579.

9. Backlar, *The Family Face of Schizophrenia*, 171-172.

10. Deveson, *Tell Me I'm Here*, 52-53.

11. Henry Flanders, Robert Crapps, and David Smith, *People of the Covenant*, Fourth edition (New York: Oxford University Press, 1996), 98-99.

12. Lynn De Spelder and Albert Strickland, *The Last Dance: Encountering Death and Dying*, Fourth edition (Mountain View, CA: Mayfield Publishing Co., 1996), 250-252.

13. Michael Leming and George Dickinson, *Understanding Dying, Death, and Bereavement*, Third edition (New York: Harcourt Brace Publishers, 1994), 494-495.

14. De Spelder and Strickland, *The Last Dance*, 252.

15. Gwen Howe, *The Reality of Schizophrenia* (London: Faber and Faber, 1991), 56.

16. De Spelder and Strickland, *The Last Dance*, 252-253.

17. Kim T. Mueser and Susan Gingerich, *Coping with Schizophrenia: A Guide for Families* (Oakland, CA: New Harbinger Publications, Inc., 1994), 233.

18. Ibid., 229.

19. J.J. Van Allmen (ed.), *A Companion to the Bible* (New York: Oxford University Press, 1958), 357.

Chapter 3

1. Helmut Thielicke, *The Waiting Father: Sermons on the Parables of Jesus* (New York: Harper and Row, 1959); Donald Juel, "The Strange Silence of the Bible," *Interpretation* 51(1) (1997), 9-10.

2. Horst Gerson, *Rembrandt Paintings* (New York: William Morrow and Co., 1968), 140,164.

3. Clea Simon, *Mad House: Growing Up in the Shadow of Mentally Ill Siblings* (New York: Doubleday, 1997), 9.

4. See Fox Butterfield, "Prisons Replace Hospitals for the Nation's Mentally Ill," *The New York Times*, March 5, 1998, A-1, 18-19.

5. Patricia Backlar, *The Family Face of Schizophrenia: Practical Counsel from America's Leading Experts* (New York: G.P. Putnam's Sons, 1994), 122.

6. Ibid., 126.

7. Mona Wasow, *The Skipping Stone: Ripple Effects of Mental Illness on the Family* (Palo Alto, CA: Science and Behavior Books, Inc., 1995), 9.

8. Robert H. Albers, *Shame: A Faith Perspective* (Binghamton, NY: The Haworth Press, 1995), 92.

9. Rebecca Woolis, *When Someone You Love Has a Mental Illness: A Handbook for Family, Friends, and Caregivers* (New York: G.P. Putnam's Sons, 1992), 169, 171.

10. Ibid., 169-171.

11. Kim T. Mueser and Susan Gingerich, *Coping with Schizophrenia: A Guide for Families* (Oakland, CA: New Harbinger Publications, Inc., 1994), 108-109.

12. Arthur Kleinman, *The Illness Narrative: Suffering, Healing, and the Human Condition* (New York: Basic Books, Inc., 1988), 185.

13. Susan Backus Brown, "A Naturalistic Study of the Ethical Orientations of Families of the Chronically Mentally Ill," (PhD diss., University of Denver, 1992), 122-124.

14. Kleinman, *The Illness Narrative,* 3-6.

15. Woolis, *When Someone You Love Has a Mental Illness,* 172-73.

16. Jeffry R. Zurheide, *When Faith Is Tested: Pastoral Responses to Suffering and Tragic Death* (Minneapolis, MN: Fortress Press, 1997), 72.

Chapter 4

1. *The News Tribune* (Tacoma, WA: October 11, 1995), B1; E. Fuller Torrey, *Surviving Schizophrenia: A Manual for Families, Consumers and Providers* (New York: Harper Collins, 1995), 2-3. See also Roslyn Carter with Susan K. Golant, *Helping Someone with Mental Illness* (New York: Random House, 1998), 55-119.

2. John M. Cannon, "Pastoral Care for Families of the Mentally Ill," *The Journal of Pastoral Care,* 64 (1990), 213-221.

3. Victoria Secunda, *When Madness Comes Home: Help and Hope for the Children, Siblings, and Partners of the Mentally Ill* (New York: Hyperion, 1997), 178-179.

4. John T. Vanderzee, *Ministry to Persons with Chronic Illnesses* (Minneapolis, MN: Augsburg, 1993), 56.

5. Ibid., 40-41.

6. Richard P. Olson and Joe Leonard, *Ministry with Families in Flux* (Louisville, KY: Westminster John Knox Press, 1990), 142-143.

7. See Stewart Govig, *Strong at the Broken Places: Persons with Disabilities and the Church* (Louisville, KY: Westminster John Knox, 1989).

8. Howard M. Spiro, Mary G. Curnen, Enid Peschel, and Deborah St. James (eds.), *Empathy and the Practice of Medicine: Beyond Pills and the Scalpel* (New Haven, CT: Yale University Press, 1993), 7, 15.

9. M.H. Abrams (Gen. ed.) *The Norton Anthology of English Literature,* Fifth Edition (New York: W.W. Norton and Company, 1986), Volume I, Meditation 17, 1107.

10. Spiro et al., *Empathy and the Practice of Medicine,* 10-11, 79.

11. Nancy Eisenberg and Janet Strayer (eds.), *Empathy and its Development* (Cambridge, MA: Cambridge University Press, 1987), 28.

12. Otto F. Wahl, *Media Madness: Public Images of Mental Illness* (New Brunswick, NJ: Rutgers University Press, 1995), 102.

13. H. Newton Maloney (ed.), *Psychology of Religion: Personalities, Problems, Possibilities* (Grand Rapids, MI: Baker Book House, 1991), 543.

14. Patricia Backlar, *The Family Face of Schizophrenia: Practical Counsel From America's Leading Experts* (New York: Putnam Books, 1994), 48.

Chapter 5

1. Herbert Anderson, *The Family and Pastoral Care* (Philadelphia: Fortress Press, 1984), 108. For discussion of causes see Torrey, *Surviving Schizophrenia*, Third Edition (New York: Harper Collins, 1995), ch. 6, 139-174.

2. Iris V. Cully and Kendig B. Cully (eds.), *Encyclopedia of Religious Education* (San Francisco: Harper and Row, 1990), 497.

3. "Power Ministries," Station KLAY, Tacoma, WA, July 27, 1997.

4. Otto Wahl, *Media Madness: Public Images of Mental Illness*, 22.

5. Rodney J. Hunter, H. Newton Maloney, Liston Mills, and John Patton, (eds.), "Silence" in *Dictionary of Pastoral Care and Counseling* (Nashville, TN: Abingdon Press, 1990), 1172-1173.

6. Stephen A. Schmidt, *Living with Chronic Illness* (Minneapolis: Augsburg Publishing House, 1989), 36.

7. P.W. Pryser, "Health and Illness," in Rodney J. Hunter, et al. (eds.), *Dictionary of Pastoral Care and Counseling*, 501-505.

8. "Morning Worship," Station KCIS sermon, Seattle, WA, September 1, 1997.

9. "Saved by Faith," KLAY, Tacoma, WA, August 24, 1997.

10. John Pilch in Jerome H. Neyrey (ed.), *The Social World of Luke/Acts: Models for Interpretation* (Peabody, MA: Hendrickson Publishers, 1991), 190.

11. For details see Stewart Govig, "Chronic Mental Illness and the Family: Contexts for Pastoral Care," *The Journal of Pastoral Care* (Winter 1993) 47(4), 405-418.

Chapter 6

1. J.J. von Allmen (ed.), "Teaching" in *A Companion to the Bible* (New York: Oxford University Press, 1958), 414.

2. Joseph A. Grassi, *Teaching the Way: Jesus, the Early Church and Today* (Washington, DC: University Press of America, 1982), 26. Advocacy for a higher teaching priority is found in Marlene Mayr (ed.), *Does the Church Really Want Religious Education?* (Birmingham, AL: Religious Education Press, 1988) and Morton Kelsey, *Can Christians Be Educated?* (Birmingham, AL: Religious Education Press, 1977).

3. D. Elton Trueblood, *The Teacher* (Nashville, TN: Broadman Press, 1980), 21.

4. Thomas H. Groome, *Sharing Faith, A Comprehensive Approach to Religious Education and Pastoral Ministry* (San Francisco: Harpers, 1991), 449; Robert Browning (ed.), *The Pastor as Religious Educator* (Birmingham, AL: Religious Education Press, 1989), 11.

5. Nancy T. Foltz, *Handbook of Adult Religious Education* (Birmingham, AL: Religious Education Press, 1986), 48.

6. Browning, *The Pastor as Religious Educator*, 2.

7. Stanley Hauerwas and John H. Westerhoff (eds.), *Schooling Christians: Holy Experiments in American Education* (Grand Rapids, MI: William B. Eerdmans, 1992), 267. For current discussion see Editorial, "The Congregation as Educator," *Religious Education*, 62(3) (Summer 1997).

8. E. Fuller Torrey, *Surviving Schizophrenia: A Manual for Families, Consumers, and Providers,* Third edition (New York: Harper Collins, 1995), 59.

Chapter 7

1. Joseph W. Alley, "Creating a Caring Congregation" in Jennifer Shifrin (ed.), *Caring Congregations: Observations and Commentary* (St. Louis, MO: Pathways to Promise, 1997), 37-38. The congregation is College Place United Methodist Church in Columbia, SC.

2. Letter to the Editor, *The Morning News Tribune*, February 3, 1988, p. A9.

3. Letter to the Editor, *The News Tribune*, October 6, 1996.

4. March 10, 1997. In a letter (March 17) the Editor responded, "You are quite right to catch this inappropriate and incorrect phrasing. Thank you for bringing it to my attention. We will change the description in all future catalogs."

5. See Gilliam Helfgott, *Love You to Bits and Pieces: Life with David Helfgott* (New York: Penguin Books, 1996).

6. Bernice Skirball and Kaye Olsen (Compeer Coordinators, Associated Ministries, Pierce County) *Meet Compeer*, Janet Leng (ed.). Monthly newsletter, Associated Ministries Vol. 29, No. 6, July/August, 1997. Tacoma, WA.

7. Ibid., p. 4.

8. Paul Reitmann and David T. Alger (Executive Director), The Interfaith Center, 1224 South "I" Street, Tacoma, WA 98405-5021. Associated Ministries represents over 200 congregations, groups, and interfaith partners in Pierce County.

9. Letter to the writer June 17, 1997; to Dr. John Huffman December 3, 1993.

10. Letter and materials from Gunnar Christiansen, June 20, 1997. See also his "Spirituality and Religious Outreach," *The Journal* 8(4), 1997 (Sacramento, CA: California Alliance for the Mentally Ill).

11. Letter and materials from Director Connie Rakitan, July 2, 1997.

12. Barbara Schneeberg, *Christian Social Action* (Washington, DC, United Methodist Church: 9(9) (October 1996), 35.

13. Ibid., p. 36.

Chapter 8

1. John M. Cannon, "Pastoral Care for Families of the Mentally Ill," *The Journal of Pastoral Care,* 54(2) (1990), 217.

2. Fred Cloud, "Pastoral Care of the Mentally Ill and Their Families: Four Perspectives with Implications for Action" (DMin Diss., Vanderbilt University, Nashville, TN, 1990), 4.

3. Spaniol, Gagne, and Koehler, *Psychological and Social Aspects of Psychiatric Disability,* 7.

4. Lewis L. Judd, "Putting Mental Health on the Nation's Health Agenda," *Hospital and Community Psychiatry,* 41(2) (February 1990) n.p.

5. Ibid.

6. See G. Fackre, "Ministry of Presence" in Hunter, Rodney J., Maloney, H. Newton, Mills, Liston O., and Patton, John (eds.), *Dictionary of Pastoral Care and Counseling* (Nashville: Abingdon Press, 1990) 950-951.

7. David A. Roozen, William McKinney, and Jackson W. Carroll (eds.), *Varieties of Religious Presence: Mission in Public Life* (New York: The Pilgrim Press, 1984), 17.

8. Abraham Heschel, *The Prophets* (New York: Harper and Row, 1962), 19.

9. Ibid., 247, 307, 313. See also Howard Clinebell, *Basic Types of Pastoral Care and Counseling* (Nashville, TN: Abingdon, 1984), 75.

10. David Hall, "Prophets" in Bruce Metzger and Michael Coogan (eds.), *The Oxford Companion to the Bible* (New York: Oxford University Press, 1993), 620-623. See also Thomas W. Gillespie, *The First Theologians: A Study in Prophecy* (Grand Rapids, MI: William B. Eerdmans, 1994).

11. Donald Capps, "The Letting Loose of Hope: Where Psychology of Religion and Pastoral Care Converge," *The Journal of Pastoral Care,* 51 (1997), 149.

12. Donald Capps, *Agents of Hope: A Pastoral Psychology* (Minneapolis, MN: Fortress Press, 1995), 98-163.

13. Kenneth J. Doka (ed.), *Disenfranchised Grief: Recognizing Hidden Sorrow* (Toronto: Lexington Books, 1989), 189.

14. Ibid., 190-193.

15. William Barclay, *A New Testament Word Book* (London: SCM Press, 1959), 83-85.

16. Harold Kushner, *When Bad Things Happen to Good People* (New York: Schocken Books, 1981.)

17. Froma Walsh and Monica McGoldrick (eds.), *Living Beyond Loss: Death in the Family* (New York: W.W. Norton, 1991), 168-173.

18. C. Welton Gaddy, *A Soul Under Siege: Surviving Clergy Depression* (Louisville, KY: Westminster John Knox Press, 1991), 162-165.

19. Leslie Newbigin, in Geiko Fahrenholz (ed.), *Partners in Life: The Handicapped and the Church* (Geneva: WCC Faith and Order Paper 89, 1979), 25. For a tale of "new day" light read about Trevor in Henri J. Nouwen, *Can You Drink the Cup?* (Notre Dame, IN: Ave Maria Press, 1996), ch. 5 "The Cup of Blessings," 63-69.

20. Marcus Borg, *Meeting Jesus Again for the First Time* (San Francisco: Harper, 1994), 121-128.

Index